GW00502658

The
Reluctant
Nazi

The
Reluctant
Nazi

Searching for
my Grandfather

GABRIELLE ROBINSON

To my husband Mike,
collaborator extraordinaire

First published 2012

The History Press
The Mill, Brimscombe Port
Stroud, Gloucestershire, GL5 2QG
www.thehistorypress.co.uk

© Gabrielle Robinson, 2012

The right of Gabrielle Robinson to be identified as the Author
of this work has been asserted in accordance with the
Copyrights, Designs and Patents Act 1988.

British Library Cataloguing in Publication Data.
A catalogue record for this book is available from the British Library.

ISBN 978 0 7524 6447 3

Typesetting and origination by The History Press
Printed in India
Manufacturing managed by Jellyfish Print Solutions Ltd

Contents

1

Oh, My God!

Corpses lie in a chapel of the Ziegelstrasse Clinic,
for the most part without clothes, men and women
together in layers.

I never wanted to write this memoir. As a child growing up in Germany in the 1950s, I heard a few family stories about the war, but mainly there was silence. We did not talk or ask about the recent past. We wanted to forget it. The stories I did hear merge in my imagination with transient memories like half-remembered dreams. I see my mother and myself on a crowded railroad station platform, jostled by hundreds of people. I am 2½ years old, hardly able to walk, wrapped in a brown double-breasted coat against the winter cold, my hands dug deep in its big pockets. From my child's-eye view I see only a wall of bags and suitcases pressing around me and more feet than I had ever noticed before. I am scared by the shrieks, sobs and shouts that fill the air. I do not understand why my mother repeats constantly, sometimes shouting above the noise all around, 'Don't let go of the suitcase handle. Never let go. Keep your little hand tightly on the handle.' She herself is loaded down with luggage and has no hand free to hold on to me. It was February 1945. We were fleeing from Berlin, having been bombed out of our apartment for the second time in two years.

Another much clearer memory comes from the winter after the war. We lived in one and a half rooms of a tiny thatched and half-timbered farmhouse in Suderburg, Lower Saxony, where my mother, grandmother and I were evacuated in 1945. The cottage did not have indoor plumbing. I remember not so much the cold and hunger of that time as the delight when farmer Ohlde, who owned the cottage, dug into the pig trough to fish out a moist morsel of a potato for me. Even better, sometimes his old mother got up from her spinning wheel to dip the potato in salt. Whenever Herr Ohlde had no handouts for me, my grandmother – I always called her Nyussi for reasons I can't remember – took me outside, past the compost heap on the right and the pigs on the left, to look for the beavers under the wood pile. Somehow we always just missed them. So Nyussi told me stories about their lives. I can still hear her melodious slightly accented German – she was a native Hungarian – and see her lively dark eyes as she began her story: 'You see, Brielchen,' a pet name invented by my grandfather, 'the beavers are just beneath where we stand now and they have warm and cosy burrows and a big larder stuffed with good things to eat.' I wondered whether perhaps they, too, enjoyed potatoes with salt. As I looked all around the wood pile for the sight of a beaver, Nyussi went on: 'The beavers do not care how cold the winter gets for they always have this cosy hide away.' I stared at the wood pile until my eyes hurt but I never spotted a single beaver. When I got too chilly, Nyussi took me back inside and I crawled under the table pretending it to be in a beaver burrow. I loved the beavers and their adventures underground. Nyussi's stories always delighted me and made me forget that I was hungry and cold. It was only much later when I was in my forties that my mother mentioned casually in a conversation that Nyussi had made up the beaver stories. There never were any beavers there at all. Even after so many years I felt a pang of sadness and loss that has not entirely left me even now.

Apart from such occasional memories, the Second World War was not part of my world and I was not bothered by the silence about it. We were all looking forward, not thinking backward. As a child I did not ask questions about the war. As an adult I realised that my mother, my only surviving relative, did not want that subject brought up. Then, sixty years after the end of the war, I made two discoveries that reawakened the past and changed everything. The first brought the war back into my world in terrifying detail; the second opened the floodgates to a torrent of questions about my grandfather, the Nazi era and my national origin.

In the summer of 2005, after my mother's death, my husband Mike and I were holidaying in her Vienna apartment. We had returned from a hike in the hills above the city, stopping at vineyards along the way. I was pleasantly tired and just wanted to relax with a book before going to bed. As I plucked *Effie Briest*, my favourite Theodor Fontane novel, from high up on the shelf of a bookcase, two small objects tumbled to the floor. I picked them up and saw that they were two notebooks bound in faded green cloth with 'AGENDA' stamped in gold at the top of each. Curious, I flipped through the pages. They were covered from top to bottom in small, pencilled writing. I immediately recognised it. It was my grandfather's hand.

Seeing his tiny, precise lettering after so many years brought back a flood of memories. I had spent the happiest years, all too few, of my childhood with him until his death in 1955. Api, as I affectionately called him, took me in when my mother could not look after me any more. My father had been killed in the war, shot down over England in 1943 in his single-engine fighter plane, and my mother worked full time in Vienna. I had been passed around, staying with an aunt, with my father's parents and, finally, in an Ursuline boarding school in Vienna where I fell ill with scarlet fever. Even though at the age of 61 he himself still was struggling to rebuild an existence in the villages and small towns of northern Germany, Api gave me a loving home and, for the rest of his life, was both father and grandfather to me.

Seeing his familiar writing again after many years, I remembered the poems he had written for me to recite and the corrections he had made on my Latin grammar. I pictured Api as I remembered him, a thin and tall man with cropped white hair who walked with a slight stoop. His bright blue eyes always seemed to be laughing. He had a fine, narrow nose and his thin lips echoed the smile in his eyes. I do not remember that Api ever raised his voice against me in anger. He invented all sorts of affectionate names for me, calling me Gabruschken, Brielchen, or his little sunshine. When we had nothing after the war, he built me a doll's house out of matchboxes with tiny doll figures made of bits of silver paper he had saved. It had a hospital where we looked after the 'sick'. Of course, I was his head nurse.

I was always happy when he joined Nyussi and me for 'the length of a cigar', wearing his white doctor's coat and filling the room with laughter and good spirits.

However much he surrounded us all with laughter and play, Api's chief concern was to teach me to become disciplined and conscientious, and to give my whole attention to whatever I was doing whether it was work or play. He had been brought up in the Prussian tradition of work and discipline, and he tried to instil these values in me as well. The only time he chastised me was when I was doing nothing, wasting time without thought or feeling. I remember one summer Sunday afternoon outside our apartment in Bevensen. I must have been 8 or 9 years old. I felt hot and lazy and none of my friends were around, so I picked up a stick and dragged it along our dark brown slatted fence listening to the rat-tat-tat it made against the wood. When Api saw this he was upset. He scolded me, not for playing or for damaging the fence, but for doing something without engagement. And then he offered to build a kite with me.

Caught up in memories, I was not tired any more. I sat down on the couch Api had bought for my mother when she got married in 1941, which somehow had survived the war, and started to read.

The diary began on 21 April 1945 in Berlin where Api, aged 57, was serving as a military doctor with the rank of major. He was stationed in the central district, what the Nazis called the Citadel, near the Reichstag, the Brandenburg Gate and Hitler's bunker. Reading the diary, the enjoyable nostalgia of life with my grandfather was almost instantly engulfed by the terror he faced day by day. He lived under the constant howling of bombs and the heavy rain of grenade splinters. Hardly a building was left standing. The familiar streets lay buried under mountains of rubble, twisted wires, burnt-out streetcars and bomb craters. Acrid smoke and dust made it impossible to breathe and transformed day into night. Together with other grey and emaciated survivors, many of them refugees from the East, Api tried to forge a path through this wilderness.

As a doctor he felt almost totally helpless to assist the wounded, sick and dying all around him. Without sanitation, and without water after they had drained the last drops from the heaters, he could not do much for them. The only light came from a few Hindenburg candles, bits of tallow in cardboard, and everyone took care to scoop up and reuse every fallen drop.

Over all hung the stench of decaying bodies and excrement. Unimaginable. He wrote:

> Just now I have been looking for spaces where one can at least have the sick sit down or lay them on the ground for the night, without doors or windows, but at least protected from rain and safe from grenade splinters, although cold without padding. Corpses lie in a chapel of the Ziegelstrasse Clinic, for the most part without clothes, men and women together in layers.

Reading late into the night I felt as if, years after his death in 1955 when I was 13, Api was there speaking directly to me, and helping me understand him much more intimately. I saw him at his most desperate, when his existence had shrunk down to paralysing anxiety with only the slenderest ray of hope to keep him going. On almost every page I also saw his love for me, his 2-year-old fatherless granddaughter, and I anxiously followed his mental and physical deterioration. Witness to daily horrors, he was driven to the point of collapse. He felt so desperately alone, unable to communicate with us where we had been evacuated. His best company was the swifts and swallows he watched circling over the ruins. They, too, had become homeless.

Finally, long after midnight, exhausted and worn out emotionally, I had to stop reading. But I resolved to translate the diaries and tell Api's story. Of course, I was aware that my grandfather was not an important historical figure, just an ordinary German who lived in central Berlin at a crucial time. Nevertheless, his experiences would, I hoped, add first-hand details to one of the most turbulent times of the twentieth century. So when we left Vienna, I carefully wrapped up the diaries and took them with me to South Bend, Indiana, where I would have time to read and transcribe them.

Back home, I set to work immediately, mostly in the evenings and on weekends for I still was Director of International Programs at Indiana University South Bend. Bit by bit I found out more about Api's life at that time. Always a writer, he had furnished an eloquent testimony of his experiences in 1945. I began to understand how his diary was an attempt to cope with the horror of war, and a refuge in the maelstrom of chaos and death. It served as a lifeline to a saner and more humane existence, a world that was all but lost. He clung to the hope that at some happier time in the future we would be able to read these notes, 'although', he admitted, 'they are paltry in relation to the shocking force of my inner experiences'.

I followed the days and weeks of Api's nightmare. The war finally ended on 9 May, but his situation did not improve. The Russians took over central Berlin and the misery, the fear and the starvation continued. The Russians, who had suffered so much at the hands of the Germans and were themselves destitute, plundered and raped their way through the ruin of a city. It was at this point, even more than during the inferno of the war, that Api was at his most desolate. Even his faith, which had always been strong, deserted him and he contemplated suicide. He was not alone in this hopelessness and despair. It got so bad that the newly installed gas lines in a suburb east of Tempelhof Airfield had to be shut down again because too many people used the gas to kill themselves.

As I worked my way through the diaries, an abbreviation kept appearing more and more frequently. They were two letters: '*Pg*'. From dim memories I recalled that this may, no, must mean '*Parteigenossen*', 'Party members'. Surely, not my grandfather? Then I made my second discovery. Api had been a *Pg*: a member of the Nazi Party, the National Socialist German Workers Party. I had not known this. It had never been mentioned in my family. I sat there with a pounding heart saying to myself over and over in the crudest and most shocking terms: 'Oh, my God, Api was a Nazi!'

2

You Made Soap out of my Aunt

To do this is to condemn your ancestors! You're going
to dig up my grandfather and hang him.

I could not go on. In tears, I could not talk about it, not even with my husband, Mike, although he is one of the most open-minded people I know. Trained as a sociologist and with a positive and problem-solving disposition, he would have been the one person I could approach about this. Yet I could not do it. I hid the green notebooks again, burying them deep in the bottom drawer of my desk. I had wanted to tell the story of the diaries for their historical value and also as a tribute to my Api who loved me and played with me, who taught me Latin and showed me how to build a kite. I had not foreseen that this supposed tribute to him would lead to a painful re-evaluation of my family, my life and my nationality.

Until now I had thought of myself not so much as a victim of war than as a lucky survivor. I was not aware, consciously at least, of the traumas the twelve years of the 1,000-year empire brought for me personally. Although I had heard about the bombings where we lost everything and about the hunger in that cruel winter after the war, it was all mainly stories

13

and dimmest memories for me. I have preserved from that time a love for potatoes with salt, but no scars. I never knew my father, but then almost all of my classmates were fatherless. There were 2 million of us half-orphans in Germany.

I grew up in convents, boarding houses, with one set of grandparents and then another, always moved from place to place until Api gave me a home. I was baptised and confirmed first Protestant, then Catholic, then Protestant again, according to where I happened to live. Out of necessity I learnt to fit in anywhere and our family's social standing gave me, despite initial poverty and hardship, a good start in life. Twice I travelled in a children's train with a cardboard sign around my neck on which someone had written the name and address of my destination. The first time I was sent south to Vienna to be with my mother and the second time I made the same trip back north to rejoin my grandparents. I dimly remember sitting on the straw-covered floor in the wagon of a goods train, which seemed to be forever shunted on one sideline or another. If the wait grew too long, the attendant who accompanied us would allow us to jump out and play. I often was scared to hurl myself down from the high wagon into the ditch below. On the second trip I somehow got lost until my grandfather finally found me in a children's bunker in Hanover. Once I saw him I did not let go of his hand until we were safely back in farmer Ohlde's cottage.

After Api's death in 1955 my transitory life began again: a boarding house on the Baltic, summers with an aunt in Munich or wherever Nyussi happened to be. When my mother remarried, I lived with her and my stepfather in Darmstadt, where I graduated from the *gymnasium* in 1962. Then we immigrated to the United States. All along, however, the silence about the war and the Nazi regime endured.

For over sixty years I had not felt implicated in any guilt. Of course, I was aware of the atrocities of the concentration camps. I had seen pictures and documentaries of the 6 million murdered Jews; the emaciated bodies; the heaps of bones, hair, teeth; men, women and children crowded into cattle cars and driven off to their deaths in gas chambers. I often could not bear to look at the images on the screen. It was all too horrible and I turned away. I have never visited any of the concentration camps. In my post-war world it was not only unimaginable but part of a history that seemed unrelated to me. In this escape from reality I was helped by the German mood of the 1950s, where everyone just wanted to forget this ever happened in our country. But I am afraid that to this day I have tried to avoid direct confrontation with the Holocaust. Even as recently as a few years ago I walked out on Roman Polanski's film *The Pianist*. Mike and I were watching the film together with a Polish couple, when I became ever more frantic at the powerful images of persecution and suffering in a concentration camp. Before I knew what I was doing, I had rushed out of the cinema. I could not bring myself to return and numbly waited in the lobby until the film was over.

When I was a graduate student at Columbia University in 1965, I was shocked to tears when a young man told me: 'You know, you made soap out of my aunt.' He was smiling as he said this and I believe he wanted to pick me up, but I only wanted to run away and not let him see my tears. I was angry, but I still felt no personal guilt about Nazi atrocities.

Yet living in the US made me experience the burden of having to admit my German background. I tried to hide it and silently agreed when people pegged me as Dutch or Scandinavian, or in the case of some with less-trained ears, even as English. I often claimed to be Austrian since my paternal grandparents were Viennese and I had lived in Vienna for several years – but that hardly improved the situation. The burden of my German origins, however, was not so much the result of guilt as of embarrassment. I felt a little like Emperor Otto III in *Dr. Faustus*, who in Thomas Mann's words 'was a prize specimen of German self-contempt and had been all his life ashamed of being German'. I have read somewhere that it is easier to avoid the patriotism which shows itself in a foolish national pride, but it is much harder to give up the kind that makes you feel ashamed for your country.

However, the discovery of Api's Nazi membership hit much closer to home. Now at last I had to confront the guilt that people thought I should have felt when I was 20. Sins of the fathers and grandfathers, going back generations, suddenly made sense. I knew little of my grandfather's life before the war and nothing about the reasons why he joined the Nazi Party. I asked myself: how I would have acted if I had lived at that time? I now felt implicated in the horrors of the Hitler regime. I may well have survived because of it. For despite the deprivations of my childhood, I also gained from the social status of my family, and how can this status be separated from my grandfather's Party association?

I played a hundred considerations back and forth in my mind. It is impossible to judge from a distance and I could not come close to imagining what it must have been like to live under a brutal totalitarian regime, cut off from the outside world. Even listening to the BBC on the radio could bring a death sentence. What choice did most people have but to watch the crimes of the government in paralysed horror, while trying to carve out their own lives as best they could? Or if there was a choice, at what cost? I could not get beyond such questions for a long time. So I continued my family's silence.

Then, over a year and a half later, on the first balmy spring day of March 2007, Mike and I drove to St Joseph, Michigan, to have breakfast at Tozzi's, our favourite coffee house near Lake Michigan. Although the fields were still brown and the trees bare, the sky was washed a transparent blue and the sun was hot on our faces. When we entered the little cafe it was empty, except for a group of middle-aged women in one corner who were celebrating a birthday. Suddenly, unexpectedly, my secret came out. I don't know why, but before I could stop the whole story just spilled forth together with my tears:

> My grandfather was a member of the Nazi Party. I had not known this. No one in my family had ever mentioned it. Of course, I cannot publish the diary. It's a betrayal of the grandfather I loved. Instead of adding another voice to a momentous moment in history, I am silenced by shame.

I further thought that it's not only a betrayal of a grandfather long dead, but of my son Benedict. I remember us looking at an old picture album when he was a teenager. He was shocked to spot my father and grandfather in Nazi air force and army uniforms with little swastikas on their badges. Brought up in the US, he had seen these uniforms only in films and then they were worn by the enemy, usually brutal Nazi men. He did not expect to see them on what were after all blood relations, members of his own family. Even Mike could not help but do a double take the first time he saw these pictures.

At that moment I fully sympathised with a cousin of historian Edward Ball, who responded angrily to Ball's project of writing about the slaves their family had owned and in the process uncovering the many cruelties and even crimes that are part of that heritage: 'To do this is to condemn your ancestors! You're going to dig up my grandfather and hang him!' He seemed to be speaking for me.

As I was surreptitiously wiping away tears with my Tozzi napkin, hoping the birthday women would not notice, Mike kept telling me:

Now you really have to write your story and the story of the diary. I had thought it interesting before but this makes it much more complex and significant. You can either walk away from this or come to terms with it. It may be easier and more convenient to ignore history than to confront it. But it is also more dangerous and no help for the future. We need to understand how ordinary people get caught up in totalitarian regimes. We need to understand the human condition in a richer and more nuanced fashion. You have to write about this. You have to get started.

For weeks I kept returning to that conversation and eventually followed Mike's advice. I dug out the diaries from my desk drawer. Although I still had doubts about releasing Api's story to public scrutiny, I thought that after all he might approve. He treasured these diaries and often mentioned that he hoped they would be read. He was thinking of us and talking to us, but he also was aware of them as historical documents and they were carefully crafted. In times of particular danger, he made certain that the diaries were in safe hands; once with Pastor Küssner, the minister of his church that lay in rubble, another time with the head nurse at the North Sanatorium where he worked for a time. Therefore, I told myself that I have reason to hope that this story, written with love, complies with my grandfather's wishes.

3

A Clash of Memories

Behind and amid all great events lie individuals, their
experiences and their actions, and it is only through
understanding these that we can fully grasp the
larger picture.

Once determined to go forward, I began to read anything I could get my hands on about the Nazi period. I acquired books about the fall of Berlin and about German guilt, and collected most of the recent publications written by the children and grandchildren of the war. Gradually I built a whole new library next to my books on drama and literary theory. It seemed to me as if many of the books I read were urging me on with my project. Writer after writer insisted on the importance of such personal stories for a fuller historical picture. Journalist and German exile Sebastian Haffner justified his own autobiographical account with the argument that 'Decisions that influence the course of history arise out of the individual experiences of thousands or millions of individuals'. Therefore, he believed that, 'by retelling my private, unimportant story I am adding an important, unrecognized facet to contemporary German and European history – more significant and more important for the future than if I were to disclose who set fire to the Reichstag ...' David Stafford's book about Berlin in 1945, subtitled

The Missing Final Chapter of World War II, added further arguments: 'Behind and amid all great events lie individuals, their experiences and their actions, and it is only through understanding these that we can fully grasp the larger picture.' Api's diaries could furnish another facet in this larger picture.

Until recently not many stories of the war from a German perspective have been published. As A.C. Grayling noted in 2006: 'The guilt felt about the Holocaust by most individual Germans of the immediate post-war generation ... for long made it impossible for them to see the catastrophe they experienced in 1945 as anything other than deserved punishment.' The passage of time, however, has changed attitudes: 'The descendants of the bombed have begun to raise their voices and ask questions about the experience of their parents and grandparents.' A reviewer of recently published books about German experiences during the war emphasised that such personal accounts are important because what we learn 'is the importance of individual historical experience that resists the either/or of victimhood'.

So now I am one of these voices. I began to think about Api in a way I had not done before, not as my grandfather who was always there to help and support me, but as a vulnerable and fearful man who had come close to total collapse and also as a member of the Nazi Party. I realised that we never talked about politics, a subject that did not seem to interest him, although it had dominated his life almost from his birth in 1888. Despite all that had happened, Api, I began to see, was a loyal German of a generation who would not have been able to share or understand the anti-German sentiments and the shame of being German that Thomas Mann attributes to Emperor Otto III. Yet everything Api treasured about his country was derided and destroyed by the Nazis. He wrote that when he saw the reality of Hitler's intentions he criticised the regime to colleagues and patients, even when it was dangerous for him to do so. In the diaries he referred to Hitler and his group only as criminals and executioners.

However, he did not leave the Party. It would have taken extraordinary courage and not only self-sacrifice, but the sacrifice of his family, to get out of the Party and risk falling into the hands of the Gestapo, the German secret police. Certainly, he paid dearly. He lost his only son and his son-in-law (my father), and his apartment and practice were destroyed by bombs. He himself only barely survived in cellars and attics, and he still tried to help others. He was, after all, a doctor; and yet he was also a Nazi.

In May and June 1945, when denunciations of former Nazis ran wild among the German population, Api often thought about this:

> Now, if such members, who were such only because they could not get out, and who more or less condemned and rejected everything in the government and spoke against it more openly than many others, if now all those should be looked upon as liable to punishment, then one is on exactly the same path of irresponsible injustice and brutality as are held against the Nazis.

He was obviously thinking about himself and I wondered why he used this displacement in relation to an imagined other group at this point. At other moments, he did talk directly about himself when he voiced his regret: 'Oh, if only we could have done something on our part against the crimes and mistakes of the government which we recognized years ago!' He had felt 'well-knowing but impotent'.

I realised that if I was to make sense of Api's life and his experiences in 1945, I needed to find out more about him. Only by putting the six terrifying months of the diary into the context of an entire life could I hope to piece together a clearer picture and perhaps answer some of the questions that kept me awake at night. Serendipitously, just around that time my stepfather brought me a wooden box, which had been in my mother's possession. When I undid the lock I found a yellowing stack of letters, documents and photographs. Many of the letters were in Api's handwriting and they covered a period from the 1920s to 1945. Several were written at the same time as the diary. Desperate to contact us, Api kept giving letters addressed to us to anyone who was leaving Berlin since there was no postal service. None of the earlier letters made it through but some of the later ones did. There also were several passports and military records, including Api's *Wehrpass*, which documents his military positions and stations in both world wars. I was particularly touched by a note Api had written me for my third birthday on 17 October 1945, in which he told me to 'Be proud and strong, devout and good to all men'.

The pictures I found in the box allowed me glimpses into the life of my grandparents. Api had lived and worked on Luisenstrasse 41 across from the famous Charité Hospital where he occasionally did surgeries. It was less than ten minutes' walk to the Brandenburg Gate and Unter den Linden with its embassies, coffee houses and famous hotels. This was the same district, now in ruins, that he later described in the diaries.

Carefully sorting the sepia-coloured pictures, I saw snapshots of family picnics and parties. They seemed larger, more flamboyant versions of what I remembered of my life with my grandparents in the early 1950s. I noticed several photographs of the family with a group of friends that must have been taken on New Year's Eve, for everyone was in costume, holding up champagne flutes and laughing into the camera. When I was with them, it was a quieter celebration with just the three of us. But we still dressed up and Nyussi helped me put together my costume. At midnight Api lit the candles on the Christmas tree and I stood beside their warm glow and recited the poem he had written for that year. They all dealt with love, peace and faith, and expressed a profound gratefulness for what we had. In one picture I am dressed up as a gypsy girl with a shiny red turban on my head. In my arms I am holding Theodor, the teddy bear a British airman had brought me from London in 1946. In another I am standing beside the lit tree in my favourite dark-blue sailor's outfit. This one, however, must have been taken at Christmas right after we came back from church and before I got to open my presents.

Picnics were another of Api's favourite leisure-time activities. Studying the pictures of the 1920s and '30s, my mind drifted to similar scenes in the sandy heath landscape of northern Germany in the 1950s. The old pictures invariably featured not only the family but whatever new Buick Api had bought. It was the chief luxury of his life. The first one, in 1926, was a boxy car with wooden spokes and a wide, curving running board. In the 1950s our pictures showed the much more modest *Grey Donkey*, a second-hand Opel Olympia. Yet Api delighted in this car. It was a sign that, in his sixties, he had once more managed to climb out of poverty. It also meant no more visiting his patients on a bike.

Reading about the Nazi era, I came back again and again to the question: why had Api joined the Nazi Party? I knew that he cherished stability and order, which Hitler promised, and I speculated that Api, a strong Lutheran, may have been attracted by Hitler's religious bearing at the time. In 1933 Hitler came across as a conservative and religious man who was committed to revive the old Prussian values Api held dear. Api fit the profile of people who joined the Party at that early stage. Like him, they tended to be older, conservative, Protestant and veterans of the First World War.

Despite such partial explanations many troubling questions remain. They are questions not only about Api's guilt but also about myself and my telling his story. How can I measure Api's personal suffering in view of the suffering of millions of innocent victims of that regime? For whatever he had to go through stands in no comparison to the agonies of Holocaust victims. And how can I even begin to discuss these questions separate from the love for my grandfather and the picture of him I have cherished all my life? I feel doubly disqualified to take this on, at once too close to Api and too removed from any similar terror. Finally, does the question of German guilt also involve me since my family may well have benefitted from Api's Nazi membership? Would I have acted differently in Api's situation? Am I responsible for 'making soap out of my aunt', as that young man in New York suggested many years ago?

This leads me to hard questions about collective guilt and political responsibility that are important for us also today. We all act politically, even by doing nothing. As Martin Luther King wrote on 16 April 1963 in his *Letter from Birmingham Jail*: 'We will have to repent in this generation not merely for the vitriolic words and actions of the bad people, but for the appalling silence of the good people.'

When I first found Api's diaries I thought I could look back over his life and tell his story. It would be a tribute to the grandfather I loved and I was glad to rescue the diaries out of their sixty-year hiding place. At the same time, I thought that this memoir would allow me to examine my own past now that I was at a period in my life where I was ready to look back. But I had barely begun this process of memory when a larger issue interfered with that intention. Api was a Nazi, and now I am forced to deal with a guilt I had not confronted throughout my life. I cannot resolve this clash of memories and memoirs, but I also can't hide from it and keep silent any longer. What I can do is raise questions and break the silence.

At the end of his detailed account of the history of slaves in his family, Edward Ball concludes: 'We're not responsible for what our ancestors did or did not do, but we're accountable for it.' By accounting and recounting, by learning more about that time and my grandfather's life, and by raising questions, perhaps I can arrive at some degree of accountability.

4

Growing Up Prussian

Work before play.

Shortly before committing suicide in 1941, the writer Stefan Zweig said about his and Api's generation in his autobiography *The World of Yesterday* that 'each one of us has been churned up in his innermost being by the almost uninterrupted volcanic eruptions of our European world'. To set Api's actions into a broader context, I had to find out how these eruptions affected him from his birth in 1888 up to 1945. Along this journey I found out that the volcanic tremors Zweig mentions still reverberate with me in the third generation.

Api was born in the pivotal year 1888 when Emperor Wilhelm I died and, after the three-month reign of Friedrich III, his son Wilhelm II ascended the throne. The succession meant more than just a changing of the guard. The death of Wilhelm I signified the end of the old Prussian era. Wilhelm I had thought of himself more as King of Prussia than Emperor of Germany. To his subjects he was the embodiment of the Prussian values of military discipline, obedience and thrift. He regarded rubber tyres on his carriages as an unnecessary luxury and refused to have hot-water baths installed in his palace. Wilhelm II, by contrast, saw himself as the leader of a new and powerful German Empire. He was a flamboyant, autocratic and truly imperial ruler of Germany. Despite his withered left arm, he loved public appearances of all sorts. Historian Christopher Clark refers to him as the first 'media monarch'. One of his favourite architectural monuments was the *Siegesallee*, the Victory Avenue in Berlin's Tiergarten, with its marble gallery of thirty-two large but undistinguished sculptures of the Hohenzollerns from the twelfth century to Emperor Wilhelm I. His dismissal of Bismarck in 1890 was just another sign that a new wind was blowing over the Reich. The emperor's absolutist and vainglorious attitude of Germany's supremacy coupled with his reactionary ideology did much to precipitate his country into the First World War, which, it can be said in turn, helped pave the way for Hitler and the Second World War.

However, in Marienwerder, where Api was born on 22 January 1888, the spirit and values of the old king still prevailed. The West Prussian town was situated on the Liwa River, 250 miles north-east of Berlin and 50 miles south of Danzig. The Weichsel River runs just over 2 miles east of the town. At the time of Api's birth Marienwerder had about 8,000 inhabitants.

Marienwerder has a war-torn history, divided between Eastern and Western influences. It was founded in 1233 by the Teutonic Knights, a German Roman Catholic military order that engaged in crusades under the direction of the pope. The knights were known as fierce fighters. Their very appearance struck terror into the native population as they swooped down on horseback and attacked whatever was in their way; their garb alone inspired fear. The knights were dressed in white cloaks that dramatically displayed a large black cross and a black eagle with red claws and beak. In order to have a stronghold against the Prussians, the original Baltic inhabitants, the knights built a castle by the side of the Liwa. They named it Mary's Holm, or Mary's Little Island, since the Virgin Mary was one of their patron saints. The castle complex still dominates the town. As a boy, Api was intrigued by a separate tower which was connected to the castle by a high bridge, supported by six tall arches like a viaduct. Api's father explained to his amazed son: 'Many hundreds of years ago this tower was the castle's bathroom. People had to walk on that long bridge to go to the bathroom. Originally the tower stood right at the water's edge, but over time the river changed course and now the tower is on dry land.'

The knights had found their match in the Prussians who, for fifty years, fought them ferociously. The Prussians were confident in their ultimate success since for centuries they had repelled any attempts to take them over. Chronicles say that they 'roasted captured brethren alive in their armour like chestnuts'. The knights retaliated by giving the Prussians the option of baptism or death, killing any resisters. In the long run that method prevailed and the knights were able to establish a sovereign monastic state from which they colonised the area. In 1330 they also erected a cathedral adjoining the castle of Mary's Holm, which became the seat of the bishops of Pomesania. Both castle and cathedral were massively constructed of red brick in the Gothic style. The reign of the Teutonic Knights lasted less than 200 years. In 1410 they were defeated in the battle of Tannenberg by a Polish-Lithuanian army and Marienwerder became a Polish fiefdom. By an accident of history, the first action Api saw in the First World War was another battle of Tannenberg, where Hindenburg defeated the Russians. During the Reformation, Marienwerder turned Lutheran and, starting in 1523, it was administered by Lutheran bishops. In 1618 the Hohenzollerns inherited the Duchy of Prussia and in 1773 Marienwerder became the administrative centre of the new district of West Prussia.

Although Marienwerder belonged to the Kingdom of Prussia, in the early nineteenth century its population still was largely Polish. But the Prussian administration saw to it that this majority was steadily reduced by a policy of enforced Germanisation. In 1871, when Bismarck forged the German Empire out of its many states, duchies and kingdoms, Marienwerder became part of the empire and the *Kulturkampf*, the cultural battle initiated by Bismarck, was directed against the remaining Catholic population. By the time Api was born, Marienwerder was over 80 per cent German and Lutheran. The Catholics were largely Polish. Today Marienwerder, now Kwidzyn, again belongs to Poland.

Api is descended from a line of artisans and small business owners that stretches back to the sixteenth century. It seems to me that the values of thrift and hard work of that class of people have been passed on to him as an unshakable inheritance. The Freses originally came from Korbach in Westphalia. In my mother's box I found a 1910 postcard of Korbach's tree-lined, triangular market place surrounded by half-timbered two-storey houses, and in the bottom right-hand corner I discovered the name Carl Frese affixed above the front door of a store. Grocer Carl probably was a relative, but I know that by 1910 Api's family had long left.

Like many people in the middle of the nineteenth century, Api's grandfather, Ferdinand Hermann Frese who was a teacher, emigrated to the rapidly developing East and settled in Marienwerder. All I have are some dates. Ferdinand was born in Korbach on 4 April 1823 and died in Marienwerder on 2 May 1909. I assume that he left his home town in the early 1840s after his father's death in 1841. Marienwerder was of a size similar to Korbach, but instead of the half-timbered construction with which he was familiar, Marienwerder's buildings were all made of rust-red brick.

Api's father, Max Frese, became a teacher like his father and stayed in Marienwerder. By then the family had become thoroughly Prussianised. The only picture I have found shows him in 1927, two years before his death, sitting in the sun by the wall of a house. He is wearing a three-piece suit and the stiff choke collar, called the *Vatermörder* (the father slayer). His hair is cropped short to well above the ears, but the very top is left longer and parted in the middle. He has a short beard. He sits a little hunched with his legs crossed at the ankles and his hands folded in his lap. He does not look at the camera but seems to be staring straight ahead. I can recognise Api's features in the shape of his head, but not in the somewhat dejected posture and expression.

Max was a staunch royalist and conservative. Although he was not himself a military man, he taught at the well-known Royal Non-Commissioned Officers School in his home town and believed in the military ethos of discipline and obedience to authority. The army was Prussia's foremost institution, its values deeply woven into the fabric of everyday life. Military parades and regimental music were an important part of the town's activities. Whether it was the dedication of a monument to the 1871 victory over the French or the emperor's birthday on 27 January, soldiers marched through Marienwerder resplendent in their Prussian-blue uniforms. The men were made taller by the shiny pointed pickle helmets, which bore the gilded Prussian eagle on top. Swords and bayonets flashed in the sun, and the population cheered and waved the black, white and red imperial flags. As the Comte de Mirabeau, an eighteenth-century statesman, put so wittily: 'Prussia isn't a country that has an army, it's an army that has a country.'

Max Frese married a young woman from the neighbouring town of Garnsee. Emma Riegamer was the daughter of a hotel owner, the Schwarze

Adler (Black Eagle), on the market square there. Api was their first child, followed by his brother Werner and sister Lisbeth. My mother had kept Api's birth certificate in her box of memorabilia. It states that he was delivered on 22 January 1888 by the midwife Karoline Toepfer. Api may have been his mother's favourite. He certainly was strongly attached to her and remained a devoted son all his life. In 1929 after Ochen, as everyone called her, was widowed and had moved to Berlin, she became a constant presence in family outings. I have pictures of her sitting up straight and unsmiling at outdoor cafes or on picnics in the Grunewald. Her white hair is combed back into a bun and she almost always wears a *jabot*, a little cascade of ruffles down the front of her blouse. Nyussi told me much later that Api never could do enough for his mother, who was quite spoilt and demanding. She thought nothing of calling them at night to say that she had a taste for champagne. Without hesitation, Api rushed over a bottle to her right away.

Api's family embraced the Prussian work ethic. Their motto was '*Erst kommt die Arbeit, dann das Vergnügen*', that is 'work before play'. Max Frese, son of a teacher and a teacher himself, believed in education as the main asset he could hand down to his children. Although his salary was not large, he made sure that all three children attended the local *gymnasium*, the highest level of secondary school, where they were taught Greek, Latin and French, as well as mathematics, science, ancient history and the German classics. Religion was the other cornerstone of the Frese family. Like the great Bismarck himself, they were Pietistic Lutherans. Max instilled in his children religious devotion and a commitment to translate the teachings of the Bible into their every thought and action. They were encouraged to be modest, self-disciplined and tolerant, and to check their hearts carefully for any slips away from these virtues. The family attended church every Sunday. Services were held in the large, red-brick cathedral, where the five of them walked along the gravesites and memorials of first the Catholic and then the Protestant bishops who lay buried there. Api's attention invariably was drawn to the three ancient stone memorials to the Grand Masters of the Teutonic Knights.

Api absorbed all this, the discipline and the devotion, the belief in education and hard work, as well as the Pietistic tendency toward introspection. They became his guiding principles to which he stuck throughout his life. As Zweig observes in *The World of Yesterday*: 'What a

man has drawn into his blood from the air of the time cannot be expelled.'
Api remained much more at home with the values of his youth and
refused to adapt to the free-spirited, pleasure-oriented ethos of Berlin in
the 'gay twenties'.

5

Seven Kilometres of
Documents

To foster men of thorough knowledge, a chivalrous
cast of mind, and an honest character.

Until my husband Mike and I visited the Berlin University Archives
in 2007, this was the limit of what I knew of Api's early life.
However, Frau Ilona Kalb, the archivist with whom I had talked
and corresponded for weeks before our departure for Germany,
assured me that she could provide additional information. There are after
all, she said, 7km of documents stored here, and she would search for
Api's employment record at the Charité, his applications and his study at
Friedrich Wilhelm University.

As soon as we reached Berlin I called the helpful archivist. Frau Kalb told
me that she had found several volumes documenting my grandfather's life,
and we could come right over to inspect them. We took the S-Bahn, the city
rail, from the busy Friedrichstrasse station to go north to find the university
archives on Eichborndamm. As we mounted the broad, stone staircase to
the station, I thought of Api's shock when he saw two officers executed there
by the SS at the end of April 1945. Their corpses were left as a 'deterrent'
to others who might not want to fight any more. Now the rebuilt station

was crowded with commuters and stalls heaped with fruit and flowers. We bought some shiny tart cherries from Hungary for our journey.

When we got off the S-Bahn at Eichborndamm, in the far north of Berlin, I was full of anticipation. We found the archives near the station, in a converted former Nazi munitions factory whose low buildings stretch for blocks along the avenue. On the outside the old red brick is left as it had been, but inside all is light, modern and functional. Its high walls have been subdivided to create ample space for the 7km of documents housed there. We were directed to the reading room, which had large windows to the south-west letting in the June sun. It was furnished with rows of modern desks in a light-coloured wood. As soon as we were settled, Frau Kalb brought us three bulky volumes, which gave off little clouds of dust as she deposited them in front of us. They were collections of letters, applications and lots of bureaucratic administrative details of the Charité and the university. Sitting by a window I began to sort through them, and found indeed much that was new to me.

Putting the materials into chronological order, I saw from one of his applications that Api started at the *gymnasium* in 1896, at the age of 9. He must have been a diligent student for he graduated early in March 1906 and was released from the dreaded oral examinations of the baccalaureate. Api wanted to become a doctor, but his family did not have the funds to send him to university. So he applied to the Emperor Wilhelm Academy for Military Doctors in Berlin. If accepted, he would be guaranteed a first-rate education, although for every semester of study he had to commit himself to one year of military service. But Api must have thought that what amounted to ten years of service was well worth the opportunity of attending this premier institution that was linked to the university and the famous Charité Hospital. While waiting to hear, Api volunteered with the Queen Augusta Guard Grenadier Regiment Number 4, stationed in Berlin Tempelhof. Ostensibly, the guards were specially chosen groups whose job it was to serve as bodyguards to the emperor, but mainly they showed off their fancy regalia in parades and on festive occasions.

I can imagine how anxiously Api waited for a reply from the academy. He knew that it was highly competitive. In 1906, the year Api applied, less than forty students were chosen from among 150 applicants from all over the country. Finally, late in the summer, he heard that he was accepted.

The archives revealed mainly facts and dates, but it is not difficult to picture how Api, a young man from the provinces, felt in the big and booming city far away from home. He must have been at once excited and forlorn. When he enrolled, the academy was still housed at Friedrichstrasse 140, near the imposing station which had been built in the 1880s as part of the rail project of the rapidly growing city. Friedrichstrasse also was Berlin's red light district. Garishly lit nightclubs and bars attracted customers of all sorts, prostitutes and street vendors wandered up and down among the throng of visitors, and there was laughter and shouting everywhere. In contrast to the vivid nightlife, by day the street looked bleak and tawdry.

In 1910 the new academy was completed, located a few blocks further north at Invalidenstrasse 48–49. It was an imposing turreted neo-baroque structure of red brick and beige stucco, topped by a steep red-tiled mansard roof. At its centre was a park. Above the main entrance shone the inscription in large gold letters: '*Scientiae, Humanitati, Patriae*', 'to Science, Humanity, Fatherland'. The academy is one of the very few buildings in Berlin Mitte which has survived the war with little damage. Mike and I could see it clearly near the River Spree when we walked up the glass cupola of the Reichstag. It now houses the Federal Ministry of Commerce and Industry and is well situated across from the new Berlin *Hauptbahnhof*, the central station.

Api never talked to me about his time at the academy, but I found a book that described the curriculum and atmosphere of the place at the time he was there. Students took courses in science and medicine as well as in philosophy and art. They had to complete one semester of riding and fencing lessons and do weapons training in a Berlin regiment. Their education ended with a course on medical ethics. The academy emphasised what Api had already learnt at home: duty, discipline, obedience and hard work. It also aimed to create a spirit of comradeship among its students. There was a *Kasino* where students could party and relax, no professors allowed. The book has a picture of Dr Kern, who was the director during Api's stay. In fact, he reminded me of Api. The picture shows a tall and thin man with a moustache who looked at once stern and appealing. He had the military bearing of a Prussian officer and the Iron Cross was affixed prominently to the choke collar of his uniform, but he also exuded warmth of character.

Dr Kern's educational vision, the book said, was to foster men 'of thorough knowledge, a chivalrous cast of mind, and an honest character'. I imagine that Api liked and respected the man.

The practical training was done at the Charité Hospital. The Charité was founded in 1710 as a pest house for plague victims, but changed to a hospice for the poor as well as an academy for military doctors when Berlin was spared an outbreak of the plague. In the eighteenth century the hospital was expanded with three large wings so that patients had plenty of fresh air and 'the bad fumes would be blown away'. Rooms faced a long, arcaded balcony where patients could recuperate out of doors. Perhaps, I thought, this is where Api learnt the healing power of fresh air. I smiled at the memories of Api walking with me in the rain: 'Notice how fresh the air smells. We may not get many hot and sunny days here in the north, but this is beautiful, too, and the fresh air will do us good.' His lesson stayed with me. I love to be outside in any weather and have a fondness for moist and foggy days.

The afternoon sun streaming in the window at the university archives brought me back to my research. By the time Api attended the Charité, it had become the medical school of Berlin's Friedrich Wilhelm University, today renamed Humboldt University, and had achieved an international reputation. Although Api no doubt was overawed by working in this illustrious place, the architecture happily reminded him of home. The Charité was built of red brick and each building featured the step gable front he knew from Marienwerder. It was a larger version of his *gymnasium* and the school where his father taught.

Like most of his fellow students, Api joined a fraternity. I know that the academy gave students the choice of three corps, but all my efforts failed to identify the one to which he belonged. All those records were destroyed in the war. All I have is his *Commersbuch*, the song book students used. It was one of the few possessions that he kept throughout the war and which I also cherished when I lived with him. The book features a mix of folk songs, patriotic songs and fraternity songs like *Oh old fraternity glory*. Whether they were in beer halls or on hikes, fraternity brothers always sang together from their *Commersbuch*. Most often the *Commersbuch* is decorated with the insignia or at least the colours of the fraternity. Here again I was unlucky, for Api's book has no such inscription which could tell me his corps.

There were, and still are, two groups of fraternities in Germany, the *Burschenschaften* and the corps. Both have developed out of the Freikorps, the freelance soldiers who fought against Napoleon. The corps tended to be more elitist and conservative. The emperor himself was a member of a corps and he was liberally toasted on each of the many drinking occasions. Corps required more fencing bouts than *Burschenschaften*, although I do not remember that Api had a *Schmiss*, the gash on his face which was regarded as a sign of distinction. I am sure, however, that he believed in the ideals of his corps. As soon as he was settled after the war he joined a club of *Alte Herren*, old gentlemen, who had been fraternity members.

Fraternity life was not much different from military life. It had strict rules and regulations about everything, from greeting a fellow member to defending one's honour. There were uniforms for special occasions and a billed cap with the fraternity colours on the band for every day. Belonging to a fraternity was a status symbol and members regarded themselves as the ideal of German manhood. They made sure to educate new recruits, foxes as they were called, to fortitude, self-control and patriotic idealism. Although there was much drinking, singing and partying, the fraternity was not merely a social club but saw itself as a school to build character; a place where a young man would learn discipline and self-control.

I imagine that, above all, Api valued the comradeship of the corps. He often talked to me about the beauty of friendship and Schiller's *Die Bürgschaft*, an ode to friendship, was one of his favourite poems. I will never forget the time when we listened together to a reading of the poem on the radio. I must have been 10 years old. The poem is set in ancient Greece where Damon is condemned to death for trying to assassinate Dionysius, the tyrant of Syracuse. His friend willingly stands in for Damon, who is supposed to relieve him in time for the execution. But all kinds of terrible obstacles loom in the way of Damon's return. Finally, people tell him to turn back – it is too late to save his friend; now he can only save his own life. Damon ignores the advice. If he cannot save his friend, he at least will die with him. He arrives just as his friend, who never doubted Damon, is being strung up, and the two embrace in tears. The tyrant is so moved that he lets both of them go, asking only to be a third in their union:

In truth, fidelity is no idle delusion,
So accept me also as your friend,
I would be – grant me this request
The third in your band!

During the reading Api stood a little behind me with his arm on my shoulder and I remember how embarrassed I was when towards the end I noticed a single tear of his fall on the polished dark wood of the radio and glisten there for the rest of the recital.

Working my way through three volumes of papers and documents, I found further information on Api's time at the academy. In 1911 he joined the regiment Freiherr Hiller von Gaertringen of the 4th Posen Regiment Number 59 to fulfil his military service requirement. It was stationed in Deutsch Eylau, an ancient town picturesquely situated on a peninsula of Lake Geserich. But I am sure the main attraction was that it was only 50km (31 miles) from his home town. On 27 May 1913 Api passed his state medical examinations and was qualified as a doctor. He then started on his ten years of service as military physician in the Deutsch Eylau garrison. He was 25 years old.

6

The Shot Heard Around
the World

... to honour medical science and to promote it
as far as was in my power; to fulfil conscientiously,
loyally, and humanely the duties of my profession
toward those who seek my help as well as toward my
colleagues.

No archives were necessary to tell me that on 28 June 1914 Api's quiet existence was blown up with the shot heard around the world. Every newspaper carried the screaming headline: 'ARCHDUKE FRANZ FERDINAND OF AUSTRIA AND HIS WIFE MURDERED BY A SERB IN SARAJEVO.' I am not certain, but suspect that Api, whose patriotism can only have been strengthened by his recent military education, was caught up in the euphoria which swept across Germany in that summer of 1914. Even non-military recluses like the philosopher Ludwig Wittgenstein and the poet Rainer Maria Rilke, who had not been particularly attached to either Germany or Austria, joined in the celebration. Looking back a few months later, Sigmund Freud wrote: 'We saw war as an opportunity for demonstrating the progress of mankind in communal feeling ... a chivalrous crusade.'

Api accompanied the 3rd Battalion of his regiment as doctor. His very first engagement – also the most spectacular – of his military career took place just over 30 miles south-east of Marienwerder and only about 18 miles from his headquarters in Deutsch Eylau. This was the battle of Tannenberg, 26–31 August 1914, where under the leadership of two Prussians, Paul von Hindenburg and his Chief of Staff Erich Ludendorff, the Russian First and Second Armies were decimated.

As I read further, I found a two-page CV Api had written after the war as part of his application for an assistantship at the Charité. It contained another revelation. Only three months into the war Api had suffered a nervous breakdown. He explained that in October 1914, while at the Eastern Front, he contracted a severe case of dysentery. This was followed by nervous complications which developed into polyneuritis and paralysis in both his legs. Api was hospitalised from October 1914 until January 1915 in the nerve station at the Charité, where just months before he had been a student. He was released in January 1915 but still had to continue outpatient treatment until June. This news was a shock. To me, a child buffeted about until I lived with him, Api had always been an unshakable tower of strength and stability. But in the course of looking into his life I increasingly came to regard him as a highly sensitive and vulnerable person. This breakdown also helped me to understand Api's anxiety in 1945 as to whether he would hold out under that terrible stress. By contrast, Nyussi, whom I had known only as a woman ailing with severe rheumatoid arthritis, turned out to be the real powerhouse in the family.

The full record of Api's service is listed in his *Wehrpass*, his military passport issued under the Third Reich. It is a field-grey document with the German eagle clutching a swastika on the front, and the same emblem appears faintly embossed on each page. I found the document among my mother's papers. The *Wehrpass* lists all his engagements and recognitions during the First World War. In July 1915 Api rejoined the 3rd Battalion that moved to Galicia, which had been conquered by the Russians. Now, combined German and Austro-Hungarian forces were pushing the Russians back again in a series of fierce skirmishes, which resulted in untold injuries and deaths. Api served in a field hospital. Most of the wounded were maimed by trench mortars, grenades and machine guns. In August 1915 Api was promoted to senior medical officer and moved to Division 101, Medical

Company 101. He was stationed for a time in Lugos on the River Timis, now Lugoj in south-eastern Hungary. It had been a Roman settlement and was then part of the Habsburg Empire. Over the next months Api was moved to various parts along the Macedonian front, which stretched from the Danube to southern Macedonia. In later life, Api occasionally thought back to places he had seen in the war, but he never spoke of the traumas which, as his breakdown shows, had deeply wounded him.

I was further surprised to learn that even on active duty Api was able to continue toward a Doctor of Medicine at Friedrich Wilhelm University, but I was told that this was not unusual at the time. In 1916, the archives showed that Api completed his dissertation on 'A Case of Bridgekolobom of the Chloroida' with a grade of A. He had to come to Berlin for the oral examination, which he likewise passed with an A. On 14 November 1916 Api was promoted to Doctor of Medicine as an ophthalmologist. The following day he took the vow 'to honor medical science and to promote it as far as was in my power; to fulfill conscientiously, loyally, and humanely the duties of my profession toward those who seek my help as well as toward my colleagues'.

Immediately after his promotion, Api was sent back to the front. In December 1916 he saw action at the Greek border and in 1917 he was once again in Macedonia. He earned the Iron Cross, both First and Second Class, for acts of bravery and leadership. The Second Class medal was by far the more common, awarded to about 5.5 million soldiers during the First World War. Only about 220,000, however, received the Iron Cross First Class. Pictures of Api in dress uniform show him proudly wearing both medals, the Second Class medal on a ribbon among others on the left side of his chest and the First Class medal pinned directly to the tunic below that. While in Greece, Api earned the Turkish Half Moon, also called the Gallipoli Star, which is much like the Iron Cross Second Class. I found this medal, a cross with the Turkish half-moon on top, in my mother's lockbox, together with the Iron Cross. In addition he had been awarded the Iron Cross for Front Line Soldiers and the Emperor Franz Josef Order. The *Wehrpass* also states that he had a medal for wounded soldiers. It was black, which signifies a one- or two-time injury. I never found out what kind of injury he suffered, unless it was related to his breakdown in 1914.

In the summer of 1918 Api was on leave in northern Yugoslavia, which then belonged to Hungary and the Austro-Hungarian Empire. That stay changed his life when he met his future wife, my grandmother Elizabeth Döhrmann. When I was with them in the 1950s, Api still fondly remembered their first meeting. He told me that he was immediately struck by her black eyes, slim figure and, most of all, by her high spirits. Erzsi, as everyone called her, was almost as tall as he was himself and she wore her hair pinned in two rolls, 'snails', at each side of her head. When she laughed he noticed the little gap between her front teeth, which made her look charming and mischievous. The middle child between two brothers, she was well able to hold her own, loved to romp about and ride, but, Api said, he soon found out that she could also stand up for herself in conversation. She was witty and highly educated, fluent in German and French, and she played the piano. Api loved music and was quite competent on the violin. So, he soon thought, in every way they would make a perfect duo.

Nyussi in turn told me that, for her, meeting Api was love at first sight. She was taken by the tall young man with the fine nose, the little moustache over rather thin lips and the deepest blue eyes she had ever seen. His dark blonde hair was shaved close to his head and, although he may have looked like a stiff Prussian officer, she soon realised that he was a romantic at heart who wrote poems to her. Language was not a problem. She spoke excellent German since her grandfather had come from northern Germany and it also was her father's daily language as an officer in the Austro-Hungarian Empire.

My mother, who loved to talk to me about her childhood holidays in Hungary, always described her mother's father, Henrik Döhrmann, as a stern and taciturn presence. I knew that he had something to do with horse breeding from the portrait of his favourite stallion that had hung in my mother's house. But I found out much more when I consulted Dr Georg Kugler, research director at the Lippizaner Museum in Vienna. Henrik Döhrmann had been a well-known hippologist, author of hundreds of articles on horse breeding, as well as a book that has been translated into French and German. The museum has records of his life and achievements. Henrik actually was born in northern Germany in 1869 but he grew up in Hungary. His father, who had emigrated from the same area, bred horses on an estate in Hungary. Henrik studied at the technical university in Vienna where he graduated with a degree in veterinary medicine. He returned to Hungary and enlisted in what Dr Kugler referred to as the Hungarian Stud Farm Department, which was a military organisation. When he became a lieutenant in 1884 he continued his studies on horse breeding at the veterinary university in Budapest. By that time his father was the deputy commander at the imperial stables in Mezőhegyes, the largest of the royal Hungarian stables from where the most important horse breeds of the Austro-Hungarian monarchy originated. It was located in the south-eastern part of Hungary near what is now the Romanian border, and not far from Lugoj, where Api had been in 1915. In 1912, then a colonel in an Imperial and Royal Hussars Regiment, Henrik became commander at Mezőhegyes. I have several pictures of him from that time. He is wearing the richly braided uniform of the Hussars with three stars on the choke collar. I cannot tell whether his hair is very closely shaved or whether he is bald, but he sports a magnificent moustache turned up at the ends.

On 11 November 1918, at the eleventh hour on the eleventh day of the eleventh month, the longed-for cease-fire was proclaimed and the First World War came to an end. One month later, in December 1918, Api returned to his regiment in Deutsch Eylau where he served once more as battalion physician, as well as in the Auxiliary Medical Hospital Number 4 in the internal medicine department. At the end of August 1919 he finally was released from military duty, having served nearly six of his ten years. Api immediately returned to Marienwerder in order to obtain a passport to Hungary and Erzsi.

In the meantime my great-grandfather's life had changed drastically. The fall of the Austro-Hungarian Empire had brought his world to an end. Hungary had to give up 60 per cent of its territories, including the area around Mezőhegyes. The imperial stables shut down and Henrik lost his position both as commander and as colonel. All at once he found himself without job and rank. Luckily, my great-grandmother Alice owned an estate around Nagykőrös, less than 40 miles south-east of Budapest. She came from landed gentry with a Habsburg-yellow house in the town. Although they had just lost a fortune in war bonds, the family still was able to live very comfortably on the lease income from their land. Pictures show her as a small, somewhat rotund person with a friendly smile. I now understood why Henrik appeared so severe. He obviously never adjusted to civilian life and to the easy-going ways on the Farago estate. In photos of the 1920s Henrik still has his straight military bearing but now he wears civilian dress, three-piece suits with high, stiff, white collars. His moustache is much smaller and he never smiles. Nevertheless, their Habsburg-yellow house on a broad street near the centre of Nagykörös became my grandparents' favourite summer holiday home. It also was Api's destination in August 1919.

The passport Api was issued in Marienwerder, a small, inconspicuous dull brown document with the German eagle embossed on its front, is something of a historic oddity. The top of the right, inside page bears the inscription 'German Empire' and beneath it 'Kingdom of Prussia'. By 1919, however, that kingdom had ceased to exist. But then, the passport was valid only for a return trip from Marienwerder to Nagykörös via Passau, between 20 August and 27 October 1919. The passport was a testimony to the chaos that reigned in West Prussia after the war. The Treaty of Versailles had ceded much of former West Prussia to Poland. Only the city of Danzig, 50 miles north of Marienwerder, was declared a free city. Its port, however, was Polish so that Poland could have access to the Baltic Sea. To complicate matters further, some districts, like that of Pomesania, which included Marienwerder, were ruled by an inter-allied commission until a plebiscite was to decide whether the district would become Polish or stay German. In the interim there was much Polish and German agitation and guerrilla fighting to win the population to their side. Finally, on 11 July 1920, the plebiscite went overwhelmingly for Marienwerder to stay German and become part of East Prussia. However, a strip of land on the east side of the Weichsel, now the Vistula River, near Marienwerder became Polish so that Poland could maintain the sovereignty over the river that was accorded it by Versailles. The town thus became an essentially Protestant German community marooned in the new Polish Republic.

The picture on the inside front cover shows Api in civilian dress: a double-breasted suit that looks too big for him adorned with a white kerchief in the left pocket. He wears a Homburg hat and still sports his thin moustache. He looks at the camera with a serious, somewhat diffident expression – fitting for someone with a passport from a vanished kingdom.

7

Track 17

In memory of the more than 50,000 Jewish citizens
of Berlin who, between October 1941 and February
1943 were deported from here by the national socialist
state to its death camps and were murdered there.

My grandparents were married on 29 September 1919 in Nagykörös when Api was 31 and Erzsi 25. Their wedding announcement said that Dr med. Herbert Frese was a retired medical officer and an assistant at the Charité. Now that he had a wife to support, Api was eager to put the war experience behind him which had brought him close to collapse. I do not know how well he succeeded in overcoming the traumas. It was not something that was talked about in our family, but letters I found alongside the 1945 diary told me how much he relied on my grandmother for emotional support and how lost he was without her. I do know that he was also determined to succeed. Falling back on his childhood lessons of discipline, thrift and hard work, Api set out to make a new civilian life for himself and support his wife in the manner to which she was accustomed.

It was an inauspicious time to build the foundation for a new life. Although Berlin still was one of Europe's foremost clinical centres, it also was a violent and chaotic place. The emperor was gone and the Weimar

Republic, under its first German President Friedrich Ebert, was powerless to prevail against the many warring political parties or deal with extremists on both the right and left. Germany had lost 2 million people in the war and 400 million were wounded. Much of the country felt betrayed by the conditions of the Versailles peace treaty, which stipulated a loss of land that amounted to about 14 per cent of Germany's territory, crippling reparations and attributed the sole responsibility for the war to Germany. Unemployment and inflation further fuelled the fires of unrest. The result was political, economic and social chaos, with almost daily reports of street shootings, assassinations and other outbreaks of violence. Most famously, Rosa Luxemburg and Karl Liebknecht, founders of the Spartakist movement (a radical socialist organisation), were assassinated in 1919 and Foreign Minister Walther Rathenau in 1922. In March 1920 Freikorps veteran organisations took over the government in the so-called Kapp Putsch. The Ebert Cabinet fled, but they had called a general strike which turned Berlin into a ghost town. The insurrection lasted not even a week. However, the anger and despair of the population was not so easily put down.

Api did not join any of the radical and often violent Freikorps veterans, but he did become a member of the *Stahlhelm* (literally 'steel helmet', which had replaced the pickle helmet in the First World War). This was another surprise in my journey to find out more about his life. As I learnt about the organisation I could see why Api might have been attracted to the group. The *Stahlhelm* was founded in 1918 and called itself the League for Front-line Soldiers. It was a conservative organisation but opposed to any form of political radicalism and violence. Their initial protocol asked to continue 'the spirit of loyal comradeship practised on the battlefield, and give mutual support regardless of social and class differences or party loyalties'. In 1925 the *Stahlhelm* campaigned for Hindenburg, of Tannenberg fame, helping him to win the election as Germany's second president. As to what party Api voted for, I can only guess that it may have been the *Deutschnationale Volkspartei*, the German National People's Party, led by Alfred Hugenberg. Its platform included a return to Christian and family values, and it appealed to the civil service and military establishments.

My grandparents found an apartment on the ground floor of a villa in the leafy suburb of Dahlem, about 3 miles south-west of the Brandenburg

Gate. I had often heard them talk nostalgically about their 'Dahlem apartment', and its beautiful surroundings of woods and lakes. I knew that it was both near the Grunewald, Berlin's favourite recreation area, and within easy reach of the city. Yet I could not picture it. So I was excited when, during our stay in Berlin in June 2007, Mike and I boarded a double-decker bus on Kurfürstendamm which took us to Dahlem. To have the best view, we climbed to the top. I noticed that in Dahlem we went down Koenigsallee where, just about exactly eighty-five years earlier, Walther Rathenau had been assassinated in June 1922 by a right-wing anti-Semitic Freikorps group.

The bus let us off at the top of Fontanestrasse and we walked for a few minutes past large villas set among huge beeches, sycamores and oaks. I wondered whether any of them had been around when my grandparents lived here. Their house at Fontanestrasse 14 was another beautiful villa of white-painted stucco with a red-tile roof. It was flanked by a particularly spectacular red beech tree on one side and a chestnut tree on the other. The dense hedge and iron fence made it hard to see much of the ground floor where my grandparents had lived, but it looked quiet, spacious and comfortable. Api must have loved the view of the trees.

It was such a lovely street; we walked a little further to its end, just a few minutes from No. 14, and reached a circular space with a little train station on one side surrounded by trees. It looked picturesque and peaceful. The station had a swooping red roof with a pointed clock tower in the middle and an arched entry way of beige stucco modelled on a castle gate. We walked through the gate and into a long, dark tunnel that was lined top to bottom with glossy yellow brick. Stairs led up to the various tracks of the S-Bahn. I knew that Api had often taken this fast connection into the city, so we went up to one of the tracks where a train was just leaving, passengers hurrying down the stairs. At the end of the hallway was a little cafe out in the open.

On our way back through the station tunnel, Mike spotted a sign that said 'to track 17'. He ran up the stairs two at a time and I had trouble catching up with him. At the top we found ourselves alone in a place surrounded by overgrown saplings and even trees. It was completely and eerily quiet. Obviously no trains left from here any more. Puzzled, we moved along the platform. Then we noticed that something was written at its edge. It was a

44

date, a number and a destination. Going further, we found many more such inscriptions etched in cast steel. Then it hit us like a punch to the stomach. These were the dates, the concentration camp destinations and the number of deportees of Berlin Jews who had been taken from that track between October 1941 and February 1943. On some of the spots visitors had left flowers, stones and even little notes.

Mike and I remained there a long time absorbing the still atmosphere so different from the terror of sixty-five years ago, when old men and small children, pregnant women and wealthy businessmen, all Germans like the rest of us, had been crowded together in cattle cars and shipped off to die. Standing on that empty platform, I was all of a sudden ambushed by the perhaps fanciful idea that this haunting track before us led to my past in a way I could not have imagined when I eagerly set out for Dahlem earlier that day. It struck me as providential that it was track 17, since seventeen is the day of my birth and 1942 fits right in the middle of the dates of deportation.

To my relief, no train had left from here on 17 October 1942. Although I recognise this as a purely selfish and sentimental emotion, I still was relieved that my birth date was not etched into the station platform with its gruesome news. I thought of all the trains that had been a defining part of my childhood. My earliest memory is of a crowded and noisy platform at Lehrter station in Berlin when we were fleeing the city. Then, when I was 5 or 6, I had been sent from Germany to Austria in the straw-covered wagon of a goods train. Trains continued to feature prominently in my life, going to and from boarding schools or travelling to stay with relatives. The happiest train rides were those daily ones from Bevensen, the small town where I lived with Api and Nyussi, to Lüneburg, where I attended the first years of the *gymnasium*. They made me feel grown up and adventurous. Then there were all those melancholy train rides into the late afternoon when I was reluctantly leaving Nyussi to return to a boarding school on the Baltic Sea. I did not, of course, think that my experience in any way compared to that of the people on track 17. My trains may have brought me to loneliness and cold, but they also led to life. Track 17 only led to a terrifying death. Still, in my mind that track of the Dahlem station, so near to where my grandparents had once lived, became a link to me, my past and my German guilt.

When we finally left the station, we noticed a plaque to the left of the building partially hidden by trees. We read:

> In memory of the more than 50,000 Jewish citizens of Berlin who, between October 1941 and February 1943 were deported from here by the national socialist state to its death camps and were murdered there.

After track 17, it was hard to bring my mind back to the early 1920s when my grandparents had lived in Dahlem. At that time even the brutal killing of Foreign Minister Walther Rathenau, just about on their doorstep, cannot have given them any idea of the murders that were to be perpetrated starting from their pretty station. I imagine that Api's mind was preoccupied with the dire economic situation and worry over how to feed his growing family. My mother was born in 1920 and my uncle in 1923. It was the time of the galloping inflation when, at its peak, a loaf of bread cost 100 trillion Marks. Such gargantuan inflation created not only economic but social chaos. Raimund Pretzel, a young journalist in Berlin at the time (after his immigration to England he wrote under the pseudonym of Sebastian Haffner), corroborates this from personal experience: 'No other nation has experienced anything comparable to the events of 1923 in Germany ... None but Germany ... has experienced the gigantic, carnival dance of death, the unending, bloody Saturnalia, in which not only money but all standards lost their value.' Age and experience counted for nothing and adventurous young people could grow wealthy one night and lose it all the next day. People who had saved lost everything, and those who had debts did well. Historians acknowledge that this went far beyond a monetary crisis. In his portrait of Berlin in the 1920s, Otto Friedrich finds that 'the fundamental quality of the disaster was a complete loss of faith in the functioning of society'. Doctors, however, were always needed and Api survived. In November 1923 the Mark finally was stabilised at 1 new Reichsmark equal to 1,000,000,000,000 former Marks.

8

Better Times

The whole nation, tired of war, actually longed only
for peace.

In the years that followed, the brief respite of the 'golden twenties',
Germany's economic situation improved dramatically. This evidently
was true also for Api. In the mid-1920s they left Dahlem for Berlin
Mitte. Their new apartment, in which they were to remain until the
end of the war, was at Luisenstrasse 41, directly across from the Charité
in the heart of Berlin's medical district. From their balcony they could see
the cupola of the Reichstag and when Mike and I were up in that newly
constructed glass cupola we caught glimpses of their reconstructed
apartment building and its red-tiled roof. Luisenstrasse is the continuation
across the River Spree of Wilhelmstrasse, Berlin's Whitehall or Pennsylvania
Avenue. Karl Marx lived on Luisenstrasse when he was a student, as did
my favourite Prussian novelist Theodor Fontane, behind whose novel *Effie
Briest* I had found Api's diaries.

I knew that the move to Luisenstrasse turned out well for Api's career but
I was to make another disturbing discovery about his relationship with the
Charité and his boss there, Privy Counsellor Greeff, director of the university
eye clinic. The sun was already low in the sky and I was just about done
with those three large volumes of documents when Frau Kalb, the archivist,

rushed into the quiet room, visibly excited. She handed me a slim booklet with 'Dr. med Herbert Frese' handwritten on the mottled-grey binding and whispered, 'I just found this. Look, it's not even been catalogued yet! You are the first to read it.'

My joy at this find soon turned to shock. The booklet contained correspondence between Api and Dr Greeff concerning Api's dismissal from the Charité, effective 30 September 1924. I did not understand. All I had ever heard was that Api and our whole family was proud of his connection to that illustrious institution. I carefully read Dr Greeff's letter, in which he said that Api was let go because he had set up his own practice while still employed at the Charité and because he had done so 'right in front of our gates'. In much longer responses Api vigorously defended his action. He claimed that the director had expressly permitted, even advised him to start a private practice so that he would not be penniless when his term as assistant ran out. It is commonly allowed, he argued, that long-time assistants can start a practice before their term is up so that they have a chance to get established. He added that the first assistant had done just that and no one had objected. So when the opportunity for a practice came up, Api jumped at it, even though Dr Greeff happened to be on holiday. He vehemently rejected the reproach that he was acting secretly. All his colleagues knew about it. Furthermore, he added, one can hardly speak of secrecy when he had put up a large sign where everyone from the Charité passed by every day. Api also said that his office hours never conflicted with his duties at the Charité. Dr Greeff grudgingly admitted that Api had mentioned something about starting a practice, but he assumed that Api was talking about some point in the future and that he would not choose Luisenstrasse, right next to the Charité, as his place of operation. This back-and-forth continued until May 1925. It may have been drawn out by some malice on the part of Dr Greeff's first assistant, who kept accusations alive and may well have been at the heart of the entire controversy.

On the long S-Bahn ride back into Berlin I remained uncertain whether Api merely had upset some people or whether he had committed a grave offense. I remember how often my mother had talked with pride about her father's association with the Charité and told me that Api conducted surgeries there. During a sleepless night at the hotel I continued to ponder what I had read. Api clearly had felt he was treated unjustly, but his arguments could not sway his boss. I considered also that in 1924 Api was already 36 years old with two small children and must have felt an urgency to strike out on his own, especially since the Charité job was about to end anyway.

The university archives had been useful, if disconcerting, but that, as I knew from Edward Ball's study of his family, was almost inevitable when one unearthed their family past. Back in South Bend I was eager to write up my findings and certain that we would have to return to retrace more of Api's steps, no matter what other surprises that might bring. In the meantime, I began to sort through family pictures. They came for the most part from the lockbox and from an album my mother had put together shortly before she died, where she had noted dates and people in her forceful and legible handwriting. Together with stories I remembered, this would, I hoped, help me to round-out a picture of Api's life in the 1920s.

Just as they had done on Fontanestrasse, from where I have a couple of rather dark pictures, my grandparents furnished the new apartment with large and comfortable leather sofas and chairs, fringed lamp shades, old-fashioned desks and tables with lacy coverings and long fringes. The parquet floors were covered in colourful oriental carpets. Two French doors with windows at the top opened from the library into the dining room. It looks cosy and warm, if a little heavy and *altväterisch* (in the style of our fathers), but the sun streamed in the tall windows to spread light.

I studied the photos more closely to look at the dark floral wallpaper and the pictures in ornate gilt frames. I still have two of Api's favourite oils, painted by the contemporary artist Adolf Hinzpeter. Born in 1879, he was an art teacher at a Berlin *gymnasium* at that time. I do not know how the two large paintings made it out of destroyed Berlin, but they have always been part of my life, first in my grandparents' home and later in my mother's. The larger one shows the Chiemsee south of Munich, a quiet scene of water, sky and reeds with the Alps rising hazily in the background; the other depicts a mountain path dominated by tall, dark-green firs. Whenever Api was at his lowest, this painting of green trees cheered him by reminding him of the many walking tours he and Nyussi had taken in 'better times'.

Api's reputation grew in the 1920s and with it his practice. He conducted surgeries at various hospitals and wrote occasional articles in medical journals. He also maintained his connection with the university eye clinic just across Friedrichstrasse, which was part of the Charité and, therefore, I assume that he operated at the Charité as well. He must have established a good reputation, since in June 1945 Professor Walther Löhlein of the university eye clinic invited Api to assist in the first post-war lectures.

Api worked hard, almost without rest. Nyussi took the children on holiday, mostly to Hungary but also to spas like Karlsbad in Western Bohemia and Bad Elster in Saxony. Api joined them for a few days at the end but only when he could find a substitute for his practice. He did, however, take time off each afternoon to have coffee with my grandmother, preferably on the balcony in the fresh air, even when it was chilly. He continued to take this little break when I was with them, appearing in his white doctor's coat, laughing and looking forward to his cigar. On weekends he found time for a picnic. I remember the childlike glee with which he planned these weekly outings for Nyussi and me when he was already in his sixties, and can imagine with what bustle and excitement they all set out; well prepared with sandwiches, looking forward to their ride in the Buick and an afternoon in the woods and lakes around Berlin. Api, no doubt, was laughing, singing and joking with the children, and Nyussi was watching the road, a little intimidated by the power and speed of the big car. Most of the pictures I have show the family on these outings. In one of them, taken in the summer of 1926, I see Api standing in a clearing in the woods, perhaps the Grunewald. He is dressed in knickerbockers and cardigan, his favourite leisure-time outfit. He leans on a walking stick and stands close behind Nyussi, who sits in the grass wearing a light blouse and little, dark bow tie. In the top left corner of the picture is the Buick with its still rather small hood and ornament. My mother stands on the running board dressed, it seems, all in white, while my Uncle Dieter nonchalantly leans against the car.

After picnics, most of the pictures are of family parties, largely New Year's Eve parties since everyone is dressed up in costumes. In one of them Api postures as a pirate and in another as a Turkish pasha. Nyussi looks fetching dressed as a man about town, her long, dark hair stuffed under a cap – yet with high-heeled T-strap shoes peaking from beneath her suit. There are about a dozen people crowded around a big table set with glasses and wine bottles and the special jam-filled doughnuts that are part of any Berlin New Year's celebration. The candles are lit on the tree, which glitters with tinsel. My mother, who is about 7, wears a pointed cap and my Uncle Dieter, at the age of 4, has a small pickle helmet on his head. I recognise Ochen front and centre, and Api's brother Werner to one side with pipe and small, rounded glasses. Nyussi is holding Api's hand and Api, who obviously just set the timer, looks expectantly at the camera. Seeing his expression triggers my memories of Api setting up a tripod in the woods when we were out together. After he had carefully adjusted everything and we were arranged to his liking, he pushed the timer which then was on a short flexible cord. He called this a *Schnippedolderich*, a nonsense word that either he had invented or perhaps remembered from his childhood, for he worked the apparatus with childish delight. Then he rushed or jumped to join us and looked at the camera with just this expression of gleeful expectancy as I saw in the New Year's Eve picture.

Letters from my mother's lockbox add information the pictures alone cannot convey. Whenever Nyussi was away, Api wrote to her every day. I am curious but will never know whether the handful of letters I now have were saved especially by my grandmother, or whether they survived by chance and somehow made it out of burning Berlin and the many moves that followed. In none of them does Api say anything about the current political battles, even though the 1920s were such a turbulent time. Instead, he summed up the sermons he had heard on Sundays or talked about what he was reading. He also told my grandmother about his patients, what operations he had performed, how he cared for complicated cases and how much money he had made. In one letter in the summer of 1927, when my grandmother was in Hungary, he told her that in one week he had earned 320 and in another 450 Reichsmarks. The following summer he mentioned that in one week he had made 100 and in the next 133 Reichsmarks, although he had not performed any operations. Statistics show that a doctor's gross income at that time was 13,741 Reichsmarks a year, and it seems that Api was somewhat above that. To see this in perspective, a secretary could expect to earn no more than 30–50 Reichsmarks per week.

Api was proud of his earnings and the comfortable life he could offer his wife and children, but he also tended to be thrifty to a fault. He was *knauserig*, penny-pinching, as they often teased him. One of the letters to Hungary gives an amusing example of this. My mother's birthday was on 24 July and for that occasion Api could not stop himself from writing: 'I enclose 20 Marks in case you want to buy something for her (but nothing silly) – I am sorry, kiss – I mean nothing that's superfluous.' He knew Nyussi was not a spendthrift and there was no point in saying this, and yet he still had to voice it. I can see Nyussi smiling as she read this all too familiar admonition. In the same letter he told her that he carefully watched his daily expenditures. His parents were staying with him at the time and, he wrote, the three of them together managed to live on 5 to 7 Reichsmarks a day so that he hoped to bring quite a bit of his weekly earnings to the bank.

Despite his growing wealth, Api lived relatively simply – his Buicks, of course, excepted. He enjoyed the country meals of his West Prussian childhood. When I was with him he still loved *Schustertunke*, or cobbler's dip, brown sauce over potatoes. In summer we had fruit soups, which I loved. There were, however, two meals of his I hated with a passion: beer soup and chopped lung. I remember sitting for hours over what I thought was an evil-smelling mess after everyone had finished and gone. Api, who didn't allow us to waste food, insisted I eat it up, although in the end he took pity on me and to my infinite relief the plate was removed. Api, however, was also in charge of many of my favourite treats. He brewed the egg liqueur at Christmas and made marzipan tarts, which he decorated with tiny flowers. In summer he made what we called 'sour milk', possible only before pasteurisation. On warm days, which did not come that often in northern Germany, he set out a large earthen bowl filled to the brim with rich, fatty milk. He carefully checked each day until the milk was thoroughly thickened, much like yoghurt today.

Apart from the car, the chief luxuries in their life were opera and theatre. All four of them regularly went to the opera on Unter den Linden and to the Deutsches Theatre on Schumannstrasse, right around the corner from their apartment, where they saw the famous productions of the illustrious director Max Reinhardt. My mother liked to talk about going to the Deutsches Theatre with her parents. She remembered the fantastic and romantic world created in such a grand style by Max Reinhardt. Especially popular was his production of Shakespeare's *A Midsummer Night's Dream*, which conjured up a magical, fairy-tale world far removed from the everyday. Reinhardt's spectacles appealed to all the senses, a fantasy world of colour, music and movement. Reinhardt, who was Jewish, fled Germany in 1933.

Since my scholarly field was modern drama, I wished I could have seen some of these famous productions. In 1986 I spent a semester as a faculty visitor at the Max Reinhardt Seminar, Vienna's academy for acting and music founded by Max Reinhardt. It is located on Penzingerstrasse just a few buildings down from our Vienna apartment. Reinhardt still is a formidable presence there and professors discussed his productions with their students. Walking the halls or enjoying the rather wild garden with a view of the Schönbrunn Castle, the summer residence of the Habsburgs, I often thought about my mother and grandparents who had actually witnessed Reinhardt's work.

One picture I found shows Api and Nyussi just before setting out for a party or performance. He is wearing a smoking jacket and she is in a straight and lacy flapper dress with an orchid pinned at her shoulder and a long necklace. I recognise the pendant. Nyussi never went out without this favourite piece of jewellery, which had been passed down in her family for centuries and now has come down to me. It is a ruby snake coiled around an emerald with emerald and ruby drops hanging from its mouth and tail. Nyussi's hair is parted in the middle and swept back into a knot at the nape of her neck, much like her mother had worn hers. I have seen only one picture in which Nyussi's hair was cut short as was the fashion. But when an even shorter cut became popular, the 'man's cut', she let her hair grow long again.

Nyussi wore slouch hats and low-waisted slim-line dresses that fell to just below the knees, and Api proudly drove his Buick, but at heart they both remained traditional and conservative, true to their small-town upbringings. It seems to me that they created for themselves an island of Wilhelminian order and values in the midst of political turmoil and the amoral trendiness of avant-garde Berlin. It was almost as if they did not want to accept that 1918 had marked the end of an epoch, that the world was changing with the speed of the new airline traffic and that they, too, were part of this turbulence.

Stefan Zweig recognised that the glitter of Berlin was covering something quite different. He saw beyond the wild gaiety and seemingly limitless freedom to discover a rather desperate desire for order and stability. Perhaps my grandparents also had an inkling of this. In his reminiscences, *The World of Yesterday*, Zweig calls Berlin 'the Babylon of the world'. He describes scenes he saw daily:

> Along the entire Kurfürstendamm powdered and rouged young men sauntered and they were not all professionals; every high school student wanted to earn some money and in the dimly lit bars one might see government officials and men of finance tenderly courting drunken soldiers without shame. Even the Rome of Suetonius had never known such orgies as the pervert balls of Berlin.

However, Zweig concluded that this orgiastic world was just a disguise beneath which 'the whole nation, tired of war, actually longed only for order, quiet, a little security, and a bourgeois life'.

9

May Day, May Day, May Day

You may call me Meier if one single enemy plane
ever enters German airspace.

Order of sorts did come, but not in any way Zweig or my grandparents could have foreseen, even in their worst nightmares.
In 1929 the world was steeped in another economic crisis,
followed by widespread unemployment. By 1932 Germany had
6.1 million unemployed, which amounted to over 40 per cent of the
workforce. Banks collapsed and the stock market had to be closed for
over a month. There were increasing strains on the newly democratic
constitutional system of the Weimar Republic and ever more reliance on the
president's emergency powers.

With manifold promises to establish peace and prosperity, Adolf
Hitler came to power on this wave of disorder and discontent. He not
only promised order and stability, he also played on German longings
for national unity. After all, Germany had been a unified country for just
over sixty years. Hitler never forgot the euphoria of the summer of 1914;
the delirious wave of patriotism and national pride which he longed to
recreate in his day. In 1932 the Nazi Party no longer attracted only radical

youth, but became legitimised in traditional circles, especially among older voters like Api. They were persuaded by Hitler's assurances, such as he made in his speech of 1 February 1933 where he outlined his Four Year Plan. He promised to replace 'turbulent instincts' with 'national discipline', to cherish 'Christianity as foundation for all our morality, and the family as germ cell of our people and our state'. Armed with these values, he promised to overcome the menace of communism, eradicate unemployment and establish peace.

At the opening of the Reichstag on 21 March 1933, when Hitler was inaugurated as chancellor, he again promised to restore both order and national pride under the auspices of Prussian values. Api may well have listened to the ceremony at the Garrison church in Potsdam, as it was broadcast in full over the radio. The cheers from the crowd around the Brandenburg Gate must have drifted up to him in nearby Luisenstrasse. In his speech Hitler, for once dressed soberly in black tails, bowed his head, both literally and figuratively, to Field Marshal Hindenburg, saying that this day demonstrated 'the marriage between the symbol of old greatness and young strength'.

Somewhere Api got a commemorative postcard of this so-called Day of Potsdam and it has survived to this day in my mother's lockbox. The card shows the Garrison church he so loved. It had the Prussian eagle on the tower and the tomb of Frederick the Great under the cupola. At the bottom of the card are the profiles of Hindenburg and Hitler, as if on a coin. The main colour effect comes from two flags draped around the two heads and wafting up to the church: the black, white and red flag of the empire, and the swastika in the same colours. The black, red and gold flag of the Weimar Republic, which goes back to the revolution of 1848, is nowhere to be seen.

Api joined the NSDAP on 1 May 1933, only six weeks after Hitler became chancellor. Some checking told me that this was a day on which many Germans from the social and professional elite became members, among them the industrialist Fritz Thyssen and the philosopher Martin Heidegger. After 1933 there was a steady decline in membership from that group, but that year the National Socialists were not regarded as an extremist party.

I will never know for certain what motivated Api to join the Nazi Party on that day, a decision which was to haunt him and which now keeps me awake at night. However, the more I learn about him and about the times, the more reasons I find for his fateful step. Alfred Hugenberg, leader of the conservative German National People's Party, which most likely was the party Api voted for, became part of Hitler's first Cabinet and his party was dissolved. This alone might have inclined Api to join. In addition, after the Day of Potsdam he may well have believed that Hitler would usher in a new era of German unity, dignity and welfare. Like everyone else, as Zweig had recognised, he was longing for order and a sense of normalcy. Or perhaps Api chiefly saw it as a matter of professional necessity, for the pressures exerted by the Nazis were both powerful and subtle, and doctors were the largest professional group to join the Party. The two chief medical organisations were being integrated into one Nazi National Social Democrat German Physicians Organization, the NSDÄB. Most of the ophthalmologists who joined the Nazi Party were of Api's generation. Born between 1880 and 1890, they had been soldiers in the First World War. Many were also members of the *Stahlhelm*, which was taken over by the Nazi Party, too. So it appears that multiple reasons drove Api to join and that he acted like many of his peers. One reason to suspect that professional considerations rather than personal conviction had been instrumental in Api's decision is that Nyussi never did become a member of the NSDAP.

Once in charge, Hitler wasted no time to weave Nazi ideology into the fabric of everyday life. *Gleichschaltung* the Nazis called it; a totalitarian co-ordination of every aspect of German life. Previous professional associations were disbanded and Nazi versions took their place. Professors, lawyers and judges were replaced with loyal Nazis, as were all upper-level administrators. In June 1935 the government altered the penal code, which really meant the dissolution of law in Germany altogether. No aspect of German life escaped the Nazis' surveillance and control. There was to be no distinction between public and private life. The individual was important only in so far as he or she contributed to the national good. Children were brought up with Nazi ideology in schools and trained in the Hitler Youth. Everything was subsumed by Party ideology. Nazi holidays replaced Christian ones so that the year was structured around Nazi celebrations: the Day of National Solidarity; the Day of the Führer; the Day of the Worker, the Farmer, the German Mother and so on. Eventually there were constant enforced charities down to minute saving plans to help with the war effort, from 'Winter Help' to the *Eintopfsonntag*, the simple stew to replace the Sunday roast. Your contributions were watched by Nazi officials from the Gestapo to the block warden. International newspapers were forbidden and the minimum penalty for listening to the BBC on the radio was twenty-five years in jail.

I know little of Api's life between 1933 and 1945. It is one of those subjects about which not much was said. I imagine, however, that, apolitical as he was, he withdrew even further into private life. Historians found this to be typical of many Germans. But I wonder how far could that have been possible? Already, on 30 June 1934 during the Night of the Long Knives, a wave of violence had swept through Berlin and other cities. Ostensibly directed against the SA, execution squads made up of the black-shirted SS, the Schutzstaffel, a Nazi military organisation under Himmler, and the Gestapo, the secret state police, hunted down and murdered everyone on the Reich's list of unwanted persons, including former chancellor Kurt von Schleicher. Grim reality must have intruded every day: signs everywhere saying 'No Jews Allowed', and Jewish businesses boarded over and shut down. So there must have been daily reminders of Nazi atrocities against Jews and other minorities, but I do not know how my grandparents reacted to any of it.

Almost one-third of all doctors disappeared from the Charité. The world-famous Professor Ferdinand Sauerbruch, who was in charge, played an equivocal role. He condemned the persecution of the Jews, which affected him so painfully among his colleagues, but at the same time he participated in a letter 'to the physicians of the world' saying that German doctors and scientists supported the NSDAP. Then again, he publicly protested the euthanasia and eugenics teaching at his institution. At one point he even speculated that Hitler may become 'the most insane criminal in the world'. Yet he accepted Nazi honours. I ask myself, how much did he know about what was happening at the very institution where he was in charge? At the Nurnberg Doctors' Trial eight physicians from the Charité were found guilty.

Although I have many photos of my grandparents from the 1920s and before, I found only a few pictures from the 1930s. The only one with Berlin in the background shows my grandmother, mother and uncle walking along Unter den Linden in 1936, the year of the Olympiad. The avenue looks bare. The beautiful linden trees are all gone, replaced by huge swastikas. I don't see the traditional picnic and party pictures, but there are several of my mother with her school friends, and one where she is posing beside the newest Buick.

On the night of 9/10 November 1938 – exactly fifteen years after Hitler's failed Beer Hall Putsch in Munich – the horror of Kristallnacht erupted: the Nazi pogrom during which hundreds of Jews were arrested, their businesses and places of worship set on fire and destroyed. Api must have had first-hand experience on the streets of central Berlin. One of the targets of this gruesome attack was the beautiful red-brick synagogue near the Hedwig's Hospital where Api did surgeries. It was only a ten-minute walk from his home.

The fateful year 1939 began with the inauguration of the New Reich Chancellery, designed by Hitler's chief architect Albert Speer. It was built in the *Einschüchterungsarchitektur*, the architecture of intimidation, favoured by the Nazis and it stood just down the street from Luisenstrasse. Its frontage on the north side of Voss Strasse was a ¼ mile long. Four square stone columns towered at the entrance and above them loomed an eagle in half-relief. The double doors inside were 17ft high, the Marble Gallery stretched for 480ft – twice the length of the Hall of Mirrors in Versailles – and 25ft of steel and concrete below was an elaborate bunker system, where Hitler committed suicide in 1945. After the war the badly damaged building was demolished by the Russians, and an apartment complex put in its place.

On 1 September 1939 Nazi Germany invaded Poland and three days later Great Britain and France declared war on Germany. Joseph Goebbels tried to inspire 'a mobilization of the mind and spirit in Germany' as there had been in 1914, but, as journalist William Shirer notes, this time there was 'no excitement, no hurrahs, no cheering'. Nevertheless, many Germans believed that Poland, not Germany, was the aggressor and they were angry at Britain and France for declaring war.

According to his *Wehrpass*, Api had already been called up as reservist medical officer in Berlin on 20 July 1939. He was 51 years old. He was assigned to hospitals but could live at home. Despite blackouts and ration cards, life in the city continued almost unchanged. 'You may call me *Meier*,' (a colloquialism which means stupid) Hermann Göring famously boasted, 'if one single enemy plane ever enters German airspace.'

10

Wedding Bells

There was a scent of disaster in the air, a feeling that
calamity lay just around the corner.

My mother attended the Staatliche Augusta Schule in Berlin
Schöneberg, a humanist *gymnasium* much like Api's high
school where they started with Latin and Greek, to which
French and English were later added. 'There was no room
for Nazi ideology,' reminisced one of my mother's classmates when
I contacted her in 2005. 'Even our art room was decorated until the end
with the forbidden, *entartete*, the degenerate, Impressionists.' Writing
about growing up in Nazi Berlin, Peter Gay, a Jewish boy, said that he
experienced no bigotry in his school. However, when I was looking with
my mother at school pictures, shortly before her death, her veined hand
pointed to a fellow student and she said: 'One day she was not there
anymore.' She had never mentioned anything like that before but I did not
dare question her, knowing how agitated she became when I brought up
the past.

My mother did not join the Bund deutscher Mädchen, or BdM, the Nazi
youth organisation for girls. She despised what she regarded as its phony
populist image of Germanic heroines and *Blut und Boden* (Blood and Soil)
love stories. She herself, with her dark hair and complexion inherited

from her Hungarian mother, looked nothing like the Nazi ideal of blonde maidenhood. No Germanic costumes and braids for her. In the photos we looked at together I could always spot her right away because she is most fashionably dressed with little ankle boots and jaunty hats, her hair cut short. Her best friends were the international 'triumvirate', as they liked to call themselves, made up of herself, a classmate from Italy and her best friend who was Greek. Although there was ever-increasing pressure to join, participation in the BdM was made mandatory only in 1939, after my mother had graduated.

As Api had learnt from his father, so he taught his children to be self-disciplined and put work before play. He also instilled in them a love of literature and music, and an appreciation of classical learning. In all of this he was more successful with my mother than with my always easy-going, playful and light-hearted Uncle Dieter. It was a schooling that stayed with my mother all her life. Until her death at age 84 she read voluminously in French, German, English and Hungarian. After her death, I found a copy of Jacques Lacan in the original French on her bedside table.

After my mother graduated in 1939 she had to fulfill her *Arbeitsdienst*, her workforce requirement. Her fluent Hungarian got her a job as secretary in the Hungarian section of the Foreign Office. Then, in the spring of 1940, she met my father, Kurt Hevler, at a *Tanztee* after work. Tea dances were popular with young people, although the Nazis denounced them as un-German. They said that the swing and jazz played there were examples of 'Jewish vagabondism', and the entire ritual of a 5 p.m. tea was British. Good Germans had coffee and cakes at 4 p.m., as did Hitler himself with great regularity in his favourite hotel, the Kaiserhof. Kurt, the son of a general in the Austrian army, had joined the air force, which after Austria's annexation in 1938 was taken over by the German Luftwaffe. No doubt the pressures of war accelerated and intensified their courtship, for they soon wanted to get married. Perhaps my mother thought of her parents who also fell in love during war and did not wait long to decide on marriage.

My parents got married on 29 September 1941, the very day of my grandparents' wedding in 1919. I have a whole album dedicated to wedding pictures. The dinner for sixteen family and friends took place at the Hotel Esplanade near the Tiergarten. The table was beautifully decorated with flowers and there were three glasses, for champagne, red and white wine, in front of each guest. My mother looks lovely in a long dress of white lace, with a gauzy veil in her dark hair that trails to the floor from a tiara-like headdress. The groom, of course, is in his blue-grey air force uniform. On his right breast is the silver Luftwaffe eagle and on his left, above his breast pocket, is the Front Flying clasp and the Iron Cross, with the Fighter Pilot's badge below it. This badge is particularly striking: it shows an eagle holding a swastika in its claws with its wings spread out over the edges of the oak leaf wreath. From the black-and-white photos I cannot tell, however, whether the wreath is bronze, silver or gold, which depended on how well he had done in pilot's training. Api wore his tailcoat and white shirt and fly, which my mother thought suited him so well. It was to be the last time in his life that he appeared in this finery. Nyussi had a high-necked dark silk dress decorated with her favourite pendant.

Kurt's Viennese parents, Maximilian and Thea Hevler, came to Berlin for the occasion. Maximilian was a small and very thin man with deeply etched features and dark eyes, which looked huge behind his thick lenses. At the end of his career he was a general in charge of supplies and I have several of his articles about this. But I think his heart was always back when, as a young lieutenant, he was stationed for four years in and around Kalinovik in the Zagorje, south of Sarajevo. He loved to talk to me about how he roamed that wild area, fitted out with a dagger, a revolver and a pickaxe. He also carried a shotgun he called a triplet, explaining to his little granddaughter, who knew nothing of such things, that it had one rifle barrel and two shotgun barrels. He once sent me a sketch of the area and included the lines he had written in what he called a memory book in Kalinovik, dated 1907, the year of his departure: 'Bare, melancholy Zagorje. For 4 years my tired feet staggered in the endless grey of barren rock. And yet, when I have sweet dreams, I want to dream of you, sunny Kalinovik.'

His wife Thea, a concert pianist, cut an imposing figure at his side. Taller than her *Mackl*, as she called him affectionately, with bright blue eyes and a halo of white hair, she looked more martial than her husband. When she was young she not only appeared in concerts but founded music courses for women. After the war she supported the family with music and language lessons.

Although marriage between a Prussian and an Austrian seemed like a union of opposites, the two families had a lot in common. Maximilian and Api both had been stationed and wounded in the Balkans during the First World War, and Nyussi, of course, had grown up under the Austro-Hungarian Empire where her father was a colonel. Both men also had married above their class; Maximilian's wife came from a wealthy industrialist family in Prague, the Stiasnys, who had lost everything at the end of the First World War. My paternal grandmother, in fact, may have been Jewish and that led her husband to lose his position some time after the annexation. I was told that he was eventually reduced to selling leather straps door to door.

My grandmother's Jewish origins were another discovery that I have not been able to verify. My mother denied it, yet when I was looking up the apartment of my paternal grandparents in Vienna, an old neighbour of theirs told me 'in secret': 'Thea was Jewish. No one was supposed to know, but we did. That's why Herr General lost his job.'

The wedding was the last big family celebration during which, although overshadowed by war, everyone tried to cling to the hope of a better future. In 1941 there had been a lull in the bombing of Berlin, which raised everyone's hopes, and yet 'there was a scent of disaster in the air, a feeling that calamity lay just around the corner'. The one person everyone missed painfully was my Uncle Dieter who, at age 18, had been drafted as a private. He was sent to the brutal Eastern Front in a tank division of the Sixth Army's Armoured Regiment. Germany's invasion of the Soviet Union had begun on 22 June 1941.

My mother's lockbox contained a postcard she had written to her brother from her honeymoon. I marvelled once again at what odd bits and pieces survive and how much that card had travelled. It had gone to the Eastern Front and back and had somehow been taken along on so many moves my mother made: out of Berlin to Suderburg and Bevensen, then Vienna, Hamburg, Darmstadt and, finally, Champaign-Urbana in Illinois. But here it was in the box and it told me that my parents spent their honeymoon at the Grand Hotel Pupp in the famous spa Karlsbad, now in the Czech Republic and recently of James Bond and *Casino Royale* fame. My mother loved the place, for in peacetime she had spent holidays there with Nyussi.

63

On a bitterly cold January day in 2008 Mike, my son Benedict and I had coffee at the Grand Hotel Pupp. The large hotel in the centre of the spa was once again restored to its glory with chandeliers and red carpet. The spa town, spread out in a deep and narrow valley along the Tepla River, was lined with fancy boutiques and, most of all, jewellery stores. We watched Russian ladies walk by in stiletto heels, wrapped in mink and sable coats. Although much of Karlsbad may outwardly look the same, it seemed worlds apart from what my mother and grandmother must have experienced.

After a short reprieve at the Pupp, my father returned to Luftflotte 3 and my mother to her parents in Berlin. On 11 December 1941 Germany declared war on the United States of America. At the beginning of the following year Api was called up to serve full time in Berlin auxiliary military hospitals – *Reservelazarette*, *RL* for short. These were set up wherever space could be found in schools, hotels and other public buildings that had not yet been destroyed. Lastly, they were moved into cellars. Nyussi and my mother were left in the apartment. Between trips to the cellar whenever there was an air-raid warning, they tried to live as normally as possible. But most of all they were waiting for mail from my Uncle Dieter in Stalingrad, and from my father stationed somewhere in France.

11

Little Noodle

One is so completely in the dark and there is nothing
that suggests in the least the end of our separation.
One just always and always has to continue to wait
and hope … at some point it has to come.

Among the letters I found in my mother's lockbox was one of the most emotionally charged of my discoveries: a stack of blue *Feldpost* envelopes held together by a ribbon. I did not recognise the tall and straight handwriting. They turned out to be letters my father had written to my mother between 1941 and 1943. Here again were the dates I had seen on track 17. These letters are the first and only direct information I have about my father. As I read, I saw that he was allowed to reveal very little of what he was doing or where he was stationed. All my mother had was a number, and that changed four times in the letters I have, indicating his reassignments. His last one was L44889A. She knew, however, that he was somewhere in northern France, not too far from Paris. All his mail came via Paris.

Except for his last posting, my father was not flying any bombing missions. As he was moved from place to place, he wrote that he never knew what the next day would bring. Sometimes he worked hectically; reading and signing orders, managing time charts, checking supply routes and working on his Messerschmitt fighter plane. At other times he waited around without anything to do; playing cards with his colleagues, writing letters or leafing through editions of the *Münchner Lesebogen*, the *Munich Reader* – these booklets of excerpts from German writers were supposed to provide distraction in the field. Often he just lay on his field bed hoping for an end to the war. He recognised weekends only by the lunch time *Volkskonzert* (the People's Concert) over the *Feldpost Radio*, which reminded him of the *Wunschkonzert*, the call-in concerts that he and my mother had heard at the very beginning of the war. Call-in concerts were popular again after the war; I remember many a Sunday afternoon as a child listening to them with Api and Nyussi. Wherever my father was stationed, he lived through almost constant air-raid warnings as RAF planes were flying missions into France. During day attacks everyone ran for shelter for 'then it thumped powerfully', but at night they just slept through the raid. Once, as he was writing to my mother, he heard a particularly heavy explosion which made him comment that 'the Tommys hit their targets pretty well after all'.

At times my father was ordered to fly for days to organise materials for the troops. As he looked down on the land below, his thoughts drifted into daydreams of how he and my mother would visit these places after the war. If he noticed a particularly pretty spot, he imagined the two of them lying together in the fragrant meadows in a world where there was no war and no separation. 'Do you think that this will ever really happen? We both have to believe in this absolutely, have to be totally convinced that this time will come. Otherwise one's entire life would be in vain and for naught.'

I was born on 17 October 1942, when the war was turning to inevitable defeat for Germany. My father saw me no more than a couple of times. He could only write admiringly of the pictures my mother sent him. He dispatched parcels with oranges (a rarity) for me and asked in each letter about his 'little noodle'. Any food he sent was most welcome because after April 1942 the most serious cuts yet in food rations had been instituted. His own reports, however, became increasingly more hopeless. I have several pictures of my father in front of his Messerschmitt 109 with my mother's name, Margit, painted on the fuselage. The single-engine, single-seater plane is hardly taller than my father, who stands on one wheel of the little plane, his hands in his pockets. He is wearing his combination suit with straps hanging from the inflatable flight vest, knee-high leather boots and his peaked hat.

Not long after I was born our family suffered a series of disasters. On 3 December 1942 Uncle Dieter's tank was hit and he sustained a lung injury. My grandparents heard from their son only when he was safely in an Erfurt military hospital. In a way he was lucky to be injured before the final encirclement of the Sixth Army in Stalingrad, what the Russians called 'the grave of German youth'. Then, on 1 March 1943, we lost our apartment when the building was hit by an incendiary bomb. This was even before the Battle of Berlin had begun in earnest. One of the few things my mother ever told me about her war experience was how Api and she had banded together with the other tenants to form a chain from the ground floor to the attic. They passed water buckets and sand from hand to hand in an effort to contain the blaze. They often had to warn each other to pat out the sparks that threatened to set them alight as well. Everyone worked feverishly in the smoke until the water supply ran out. Luckily, no one was hurt, but the apartment was completely destroyed. I had been told later that we eventually found another place to live, but never knew the location except that it was also in Berlin Mitte and close to Luisenstrasse, and that it, too, was destroyed by a bomb.

It was becoming all too clear that by 1943 the German air force was completely overtaxed and under-equipped. Hitler had steadfastly refused to develop new aeroplanes, in contrast to the Allies who did so with great success. Nor were there enough experienced pilots left and none of them, my father included, had experience in dropping bombs. Nevertheless, in mid-1943 Hitler ordered the resumption of bomb attacks against England with the aim of damaging the take-off and landing places of RAF bombers. This meant that planes which had not been intended for bombing missions had to be fitted out for them.

On what was to be his last reassignment, starting in April 1943, my father was stationed in a castle somewhere in France. He had time to write almost daily since they were flying training missions by day, but could rest at night. My father missed his former comrades with whom he had become close and felt a stranger in his new surroundings. He had been a member of *Schnellkampfgeschwader* 10, stationed in Cognac, France, where there was a large contingent of Luftflotte 3. He was learning to fly the Fw 190, the Focke-Wulf plane called the *Würger*, the Shrike. Like the Messerschmitt 109 on which he had trained this was a single-seat, single-engine plane, but it was the powerhouse of the fighter planes which could fly ground attacks, serve as long-range bomber escort and as night-fighter. The lessons he took included formation flying, air-to-ground firing and bombing training.

Throughout the spring of 1943 my father tried to get telephone connections to Berlin, but for the most part could not get through. So he wrote letter after letter expressing his worry about what was happening there and how we dealt with the air raids. When he wrote again on 15 May 1943, he realised only when he was almost finished that it was Mother's Day. He had forgotten all about it, but he promised that he would rush out immediately to buy flowers and decorate my mother's and my picture with them. Then, less than two weeks before his death, he wrote:

> But one is so completely in the dark and there is nothing that suggests in the least the end of our separation. One just always and always has to continue to wait and hope … at some point it has to come.

Reading this, I understand why the Lale Andersen song '*Es geht alles vorüber, es geht alles vorbei*' had been so popular. So many people must have shared the hope of the song that 'All will be over, all goes away'. As it was, most of my parents' brief marriage was by correspondence.

His last blue *Feldpost* envelope bears a stamp with a special message urging women to volunteer to work in the Post Office: 'Women and girls report to help at the Reich Post. It connects front and homeland.' Inside is only a scrap of paper. My father hastily informed my mother that he could not give specific information about his future except to say that 'very shortly it will start and that it's directed toward England'. My mother told me later that my father was well aware that his missions had become suicidal. It was obvious to him and his colleagues. The plane had to carry a 550lb bomb and a 66-gallon drop fuel tank in order to fly longer distances. General Theo Osterkamp of the Luftwaffe saw it 'as completely insane to hang bombs under the bellies of my fighters'. As a result of the extra weight the planes were slow, had difficulty reaching even 5,000m in height and were hard to manoeuvre. The swimming vest, oxygen mask and parachute were hardly enough to save the pilot. The instructions for their 'tip and run' missions were to fly very low near their target to get under the British radar, quickly drop their bombs and hurry back to safety.

One of the most emotional pieces of information from that lockbox is a letter from Captain Schumann, dated 5 June 1943. He wrote to my mother to say that her husband had not returned from their mission of 4 June to the town of Eastbourne on the south-east coast of England, and that he had to be counted as missing at this point. Kurt, he explained, was his *Rottenflieger*, or wing man, and I found out that in the two-man formation, called a *Rotte*, the wing man flies behind and to the side of the leader:

> At our destination we came under intense anti aircraft fire. We were no more than 20–30 meters high! Kurt probably got a direct hit on his engine since a trail of black smoke poured out from behind. He was last seen when, already at an altitude of 250–300 meters, he veered off over the English mainland, probably just about ready to bail out. We all hope that this supposition is correct, for in the short time we have been together we all have got to know Kurt as a dear and honest colleague whose loss would hit us very hard.

My father's plane crashed over Bexhill-on-Sea on 4 June 1943. Effective 1 June 1943 he was promoted from *Oberleutnant*, Flying Officer, to *Hauptmann*, Flight Lieutenant.

The *Kriegstagebuch des Oberkommandos der Wehrmacht* (the *War Diary of the Armed Forces Chief Command*, OKW for short), which gave daily logs and summaries of activities, had just one sentence for Luftflotte 3 over England on 4 June 1943: '11:27 attack on Eastbourne by 15 FW 190.'

My father is buried in Cannock Chase, Staffordshire. I went to visit the large military cemetery in 1967, shortly after its opening – the result of a collaboration between the German War Graves Commission and the Commonwealth War Graves Commission. The cemetery lies in a quiet valley of birch and pine trees, far from the noise of traffic and the bustle of Birmingham. As I looked over the hundreds of markers, where close to

5,000 German servicemen from both wars are buried, I despaired of ever finding my father's grave. An old attendant was walking among the stones. Hesitantly, I asked him about Captain Kurt Hevler, a fighter pilot. His eyes lit up as if I had inquired about an old friend. Without hesitation he took me to one of the rough-hewn granite stones deep in heather. And there it was; my father's grave with his name engraved on the stone. The attendant stood with me. We talked a little and he knew all the names in this section where many other fighter pilots lie buried. He talked about their bravery and how they deserved this quiet resting place. To him they were no longer enemies who just over thirty years ago had dropped bombs on his country and, judging by his age, he most likely had served in the war himself. Now he tended his former enemies' graves with love and care. He was glad I had come and that we could share this peaceful moment together. I was moved to tears by the kindness and compassion of that old man even more than by the gravesite of a father I had never known.

12

Christmas Trees

An overture to the play about hell which yet always
delighted again.

The Battle for Berlin began in November 1943. 'No other Second
World War bombing campaign against a single target was pressed
so hard, for so long and at such cost as the attempt to destroy
Berlin.' Sir Arthur Harris, marshal of the Royal Air Force and
head of Bomber Command, had high hopes that it would bring Germany
to its knees. He predicted that the Battle of Berlin 'will cost us between 400
and 500 aircraft. It will cost Germany the war.' Altogether, he ordered an
incredible 14,562 sorties over Berlin. The raids destroyed much of central
Berlin, killing thousands of Berliners and rendering hundreds of thousands
homeless. Yet they failed to provide the knockout blow Bomber Harris had
hoped for. The attacks concentrated on the centre of Berlin and by 1944
hardly a house was undamaged. An observer riding the *Stadtbahn* wrote in
March 1944 that 'from Alexanderplatz to the Zoo you can see nothing but
ruins ... Despite this they all try to live in the ruins and cellars, dirty, sick and
desperate, or rather apathetic and stupid'.

Like all Berliners, my family established an eerie routine around the
clockwork bomb attacks. Life was scheduled around radio announcements,
which reported enemy planes and air raids, and everyone got used to the

military terminology: '*Achtung, Achtung. Wir geben eine Luftlagemeldung,*' 'Attention. Attention. Here follows a message about air space.' Or '*Achtung, Achtung. Gefechtsstand der Flakdivision Berlin,*' 'Attention. Attention. Combat situation of Flak Division Berlin.' The howl of sirens, swelling and subsiding three times, made everyone scramble for shelter. You had ten minutes between the first alarm and the attack. People scampered out of buses and streetcars, looking for the nearest bomb shelter; they ran down stairs of apartment buildings clutching a few treasured items, and a suitcase or two always stood ready at the door for these daily descents. Secretaries grabbed their typewriters and bundles of papers, trying to carry on business as usual, and hospital staff manoeuvred patients into medical cellars. Thousands sheltered in the S-Bahn tunnels under the huge dome of Anhalter station. Only a few people, either fearless or too apathetic to care any longer what happened to them, stayed where they were and waited the attack out. The city suddenly was a ghost town, empty of people and traffic. Then came the droning of planes just above roof level, the whistle and hiss of the bombs followed by the 'boom boom boom' of explosions and the staccato hammering of anti-aircraft missiles.

Even if one's building was spared a direct hit it shook and groaned, windows and doors were splintered by the air pressure, and debris rained down in the cellar. With a hit nearby, it got worse. Marianne Mackinnon describes what she experienced when the building across the street from her was demolished:

> A gargantuan force lifts us off the floor, dumps us again. Heads and bodies crash against each other in the dark, my ear drums stretch painfully. With no time to scream, I am ready to be absorbed by an infinite darkness or to step into a radiant light ... But only mortar crumbles from the walls and dust quickly fills the cellar. Hands and feet fumble around, people gasp for air, children find their voices ... And now, half blind and coughing, we do not wait for the all clear, but follow the beam and the warden's reassuring voice, holding on to each other's sleeves or coat tails, stumbling up the dust-clogged cellar staircase amid choking and spitting noises ... the main entrance door has been blasted inside, and the view across the street is laid bare: a

mound of rubble and twisted steel steaming with dust in the light of a gauze-veiled moon ...

The horror of the Hamburg firestorm in July 1943, which was part of the RAF Operation Gomorrah, had taught Berlin a terrifying lesson. Overnight half of the city of Hamburg fell into ashes. After the raids were over, the fires burnt so fiercely that the city became like one huge oven that sucked up the air, creating a hurricane and a smoke column 7,000m in height. It sounded like a thundering train as gale-force winds fanned the flames into an inferno of heat. People instantly were shrivelled into charred skeletons no larger than a small child, or burned to death even in their shelters.

After the Hamburg firestorm Berlin prepared to make the city as fireproof as possible. Each larger building was assigned an air-raid warden, who saw to it that tenants made the necessary preparations. There had to be a complete blackout of all windows and in each apartment people had to roll up their carpets, take down curtains and move upholstery into the middle of the room, away from windows. Most importantly, a supply of sand and water had to be on hand to squelch the firebombs before they could spread. Sand was delivered to every street in the inner city from where people were to carry it in buckets up to their attics. All cellars had to be made into air-raid shelters with holes broken through connecting walls so that people would not be trapped when a cellar room collapsed. Attics had to be bare, stripped of all debris and any partitions broken down so that firebombs could be reached immediately and choked with sand.

Conditions in bunkers grew ever worse. They were damp, dusty, dark and overcrowded. Whenever possible my mother took me to the Charité bunker, which was in better shape than the Luisenstrasse cellar. My mother told me that I, just over 1 year old, was not much bothered by any of this. She said that I clapped my hands saying 'Boom!' whenever I heard an attack.

At night the sky was lit by marker bombs, popularly known as 'Christmas trees' because of their red, yellow and green cascades of light that slowly spread as they drifted to earth. The beautiful spectacle identified bombing targets, 'an overture to the play about hell which yet always delighted again'. Berliners, known for their sarcastic wit, joked that the situation was not critical until you could reach the front by underground. The Battle of Berlin was costly not only to civilian life in Berlin, but also to the RAF, which lost 2,690 crew members and 625 bomber planes – chiefly four-engine Lancasters which carried a 22,000lb bomb known as the 'Grand Slam'.

In October 1943 Api had been promoted from *Hauptmann* to *Oberstabsarzt* in reserve with the rank of major. Next to surgeons, eye doctors were in special demand because of the many eye injuries caused by flying shrapnel. He served in an auxiliary military clinic in Berlin Steglitz, directly south of the centre. In January 1944 he earned the *Kriegsverdienstkreuz*, the War Merit Cross, for acts of bravery not directly connected to front-line action.

One of the very worst air raids occurred on 3 February 1945 when American B-17 bombers, the Flying Fortresses of the 8th Air Force, dropped 2,272 tons of bombs on the centre of Berlin, creating two 1-mile-high smoke columns. This was probably the one where we lost our second apartment and that convinced Api that Nyussi, my mother and I had to leave Berlin. Thinking about where we could go, it made no sense to flee to the East since the Russians already were driving thousands of refugees west toward Berlin, but Nyussi had distant relatives in Lower Saxony, about 160 miles north-west of Berlin, from where her grandfather had emigrated to Hungary. Once again the lockbox helped with information here, a torn and creased piece of paper headed '*Abreisebescheinigung*', 'certificate of departure'. I was astounded that even at this eleventh hour German bureaucracy was still churning away. I should not have been all that surprised, since as late as April 1945 the mayor of Berlin announced that no new dog licences would be issued this year and the old ones remained valid!

My mother had talked to me once about our harrowing journey in an overcrowded train that stopped often because of bomb attacks. We were headed to the district town Uelzen, near where our relatives had their farm in the tiny village of Holxen. I am unsure whether what I remember is her story about this trip rather than the actual station platform in Berlin and my mother's urgent admonition to hold on to the suitcase. That long journey was the first of many train trips I was to take in the next years, most of them by myself. It was 6 February 1945, just a few weeks before the 18 March proclamation for all women and children to leave the city. None of us, Nyussi, my mother or I, would ever live in Berlin again.

13

Unwelcome Guests

At least I know my next move.

Nyussi, my mother and I were assigned to one and a half rooms in a small, thatched farmhouse belonging to the Ohlde family in Suderburg, less than 2 miles from Holxen where our relatives the Steinkes lived. We could not stay with them since their house already was overcrowded with refugees. The Ohldes were poor, had no land of their own and made a sparse living with chickens, bees, a couple of pigs and a sheep for wool. Their cottage stood right at the end of the village, next to the cemetery with its huge old oak trees. We were not welcome guests. The family was forced into giving up space to us city strangers when they had hardly room enough for farmer Ohlde, his wife, their daughter and Herr Ohlde's mother. At first we could hardly communicate with the family. They spoke the Low German dialect, *Plattdeutsch*, which is closely related to Dutch and English. But I soon learned to speak *Plattdeutsch* like the locals.

Altogether, the villagers of Suderburg were not happy about all the refugees crowding their homes, especially since they were all big city people. The cottage next to us housed refugees from the Hamburg bombings. It belonged to the Klapproth family who, like the Ohldes, were poor. The father served as both church warden and gravedigger. One of his jobs was to ring the bells of the ancient Suderburg church. Hearing the church bells toll in the evening or on Sunday, we always thought of old Herr Klapproth up there in the medieval tower pulling the bell ropes.

The Ohlde's cottage was primitive. The low entry door gave on to a dark, narrow corridor which led to the kitchen in the back of the house. When they were not working outside, the Ohldes spent most of their time there. To the left of the entry was the *gute Stube*, the fancy parlour, which was rarely used except for the spinning wheel belonging to farmer Ohlde's mother. To the right of the entrance were our rooms, the larger was no more than 10ft x 10ft, and the smaller one had just enough space for a bed and dresser. That room was especially cold with thick mould growing on its two outside walls. There was a stove in the larger room but often we had nothing with which to heat it. Its two windows looked out on to a sandy road and fields beyond with a wooded hill in the distance, the *Blauer Berg*, the Blue Mountain. The bedroom window gave on to the village cemetery. 'At least I know my next move,' quipped my always witty grandmother. She and I slept in that little room while my mother had to make do with some blankets for a makeshift bed in the outer room.

The old farmhouse had no indoor plumbing. The outhouse was in the back, across the unpaved farmyard and past the pigsty on the left. It had a little heart-shaped hole in the rickety wooden door. To the right was an enormous compost heap. Chickens and a rooster scratched in the sand of the yard. At the very back were a vegetable patch and farmer Ohlde's beehives. Water had to be fetched from a well in the backyard. I loved to help pump the water with the big, curved iron handle that always squeaked so noisily.

The Steinkes gave us a little electric cooker on which my mother prepared our watery soups and heated the chicory coffee we called *Muckefuck*. The term, I learned later, had been used since the Franco-Prussian wars of 1870–71. It derives from the French *Mocca faux*, or false coffee. For Germans, *Muckefuck* is any variety of substitute coffee made from grain or chicory. Even with donations from our relatives, food always was a problem. Although both Nyussi and my mother made sure I got more than they did themselves, I was always hungry. Nyussi thought up ever-new ways to distract me from my misery. When we weren't out looking for the beavers, she told me stories and invented adventures for my doll. On Sundays we walked together to the ancient village church. It was built of red brick and timber, like most of the houses of the area, but its tower stuck out incongruously. Round and squat, barely taller than the church itself, it was constructed of rough grey field stones. The tower dates back to 1003, the last remnant of a castle, the Suder castle, after which the village was named. Its little pointed roof decked in red tiles had been added much later. The small church had three long and narrow white-framed windows on each side.

Unlike the inferno of the Berlin we had left behind, here everything was quiet, almost eerily so, as if there was no war. Farmer Ohlde fed his chickens and pigs – although he had some trouble with these chores as all the fingers on his right hand were missing two joints where a circular saw had cut them off – and his wife planted cabbage, carrots, potatoes and peas, just as she had done in peacetime.

14

A Death in Prague

It will be wonderful when I can help so that you can
enjoy peace after a rather agitated life (even I begin
to think of mine that way) in a way you have always
desired. And that will happen – dead certain.

The first entry in Api's green diary is just one word, 'Prag'. Prag
is underscored painfully hard several times and below it is a
pencilled iron cross. The date is 14 February 1945. It is the day my
Uncle Dieter was killed during an air raid on the Charles Bridge in
Prague. We had left Berlin just over a week before, so Api was alone when a
telegram told him of the death of his only son. He was working in the large
auxiliary military clinic, RL 122, set up in an industrial building of Berlin
Tempelhof. Except for a few lists and a brief note, Api wrote nothing more in
the diary until 21 April 1945.

Dieter had survived Russia: first the heat of the steppes, then the rain and
mud, and finally the snow and ice. He had written how they had not enough
warm clothing and not enough food, but more than enough lice, fleas, ticks
and mice. He was among the endless lines of Tiger tanks that were the first to
reach Stalingrad, a big industrial city that stretched for miles on the western
bank of the Volga River. For weeks he had been stationed on the river north
of the city, sleeping in a large hole under his tank. Stalingrad was completely

destroyed by the Germans before they in turn were annihilated. Vasily Grossmann, who was following General Zhukov, described the destruction in these words: 'Stalingrad is burned down. Stalingrad is in ashes. It is dead.' But Dieter had survived Stalingrad, only to be killed by a stray bomb almost at the end of the war.

Two letters of my Uncle Dieter's, which both Api and Nyussi had read so often they almost had memorised them, helped me to understand the depth of their loss as well as the changes the war had wrought in my previously carefree uncle. Both were written from Prague and my grandparents had carefully preserved them – after his death they even typed copies of them. One was dated 3 December 1944, exactly two years after Dieter had been wounded in Stalingrad. Part of the letter says:

> The war has taught us to ignore appearances. In my mind an inner connectedness appears far more beautiful than a mere physical existence side by side. Such thoughts could – I believe – make it easier to bear even an eternal separation.

His words seemed both like a premonition of death and an attempt to console his parents by telling them that their bond went beyond physical presence. In the same letter, Dieter also assured my mother that she was not to worry about her and my future for he was going to take care of us. He himself was only 22 years old.

In the other letter Dieter wrote that he was looking forward to the moment when he would be able to express his gratitude in more than words:

> It will be wonderful when I can help so that you can enjoy peace after a rather agitated life (even I begin to think of mine that way) in a way you have always desired. And that will happen – dead certain.

That 'dead certain', however, written only weeks before his death, must have struck them as a particularly ghastly irony.

Over the weeks following this dreadful news Api fell ill. I found a yellowed and creased document in my mother's box which said that Api was unfit for duty and had been granted sick leave from 11 March until 10 April 1945. It seems that after his son's death Api had suffered a nervous collapse, somewhat like the one that struck him down at the beginning of the First World War. Seeing that partly torn and folded bit of paper, I realised how precarious things had become by that time. The troop physician's certificate was handwritten on the back of some official form and hand-stamped at the top 'Army Commander Troop Physician'.

Dieter's remains have recently been transferred to a newly established war cemetery outside Cheb. He is buried in a grave with four other fallen men. The simple stone cross shows that two of them are unknown soldiers.

15

Leave

My silly exaggerated sense of duty.

Api's next entry comes on 10 March 1945. It is a single letter, a 'U', written in bold over a list of errands and people to see. The 'U' stands for *Urlaub*, or leave, in anticipation of his trip to see us the following day. Beneath it, feeling already closer to Nyussi, he added in Hungarian 'one more day and then the one single uniquely fortunate day'. Api's diary is silent about that month in Suderburg but I can piece together the main events from memories he recorded when he was back in Berlin, from his letters and, now for the first time here, also from my own memory.

Api had been unable to send us word of his imminent arrival. On Sunday evening, 11 March, he knocked on one of the low windows of our room. We were just sitting down to a meagre dinner. Api was pale and tired from the long journey, his major's uniform dusty and crumpled, but despite fatigue and hunger his eyes shone with anticipation. It was the happiest reunion, he wrote later, although we could celebrate only with nettle soup made from the dense stand of nettles that lined the road.

Even though we had little and were crammed into a tiny and cold space, Api relished the days that we were together. We gathered wood and what Api called *Schuckchen*, pine cones, for the stove from the forests around.

They were not easy to find since other refugees were hunting for them as well. On clear evenings Api, always intent on my learning new things, took me outside to study the night sky and point out the constellations. When we came back the grown ups gathered around the table to play cards and drink *Muckefuck*. As they were settling down I went to bed in the little room, curling up in the middle of the bed so that my grandparents would have room on either side of me.

One of Api's first actions was to ask the minister whether we could hang a funeral wreath for my Uncle Dieter in his church. He readily agreed and every Sunday on entering Api always greeted the spot between the north windows, and we tried to sit near it during services.

The day of departure came all too soon. On Monday evening, 9 April, Api took a last stroll arm in arm with Nyussi, trying, once again, to discuss what to do. As they walked on the sandy path outside the farmhouse, they looked at the Blue Mountain to the south. In the four weeks Api had stayed with us he had come to love that tranquil vista, and in days to come he would often think back nostalgically to our Blue Mountain. It was not really a mountain at all, just a small hill that rose out of the fields across from the swift-moving Hardau creek where my mother rinsed our washing until her hands bled from the cold. The mist that was part of the northern German climate made the hill shimmer in a pale blue light. The road skirted the oak-darkened cemetery, and they could just make out where it curved up a mild incline to the village of Holxen and the big farmhouse of Nyussi's relatives the Steinkes.

The air was heavy and moist as it always was in this northern part of the country, even in summer. Nyussi could not get used to the constant dampness and fog. Her hands and feet were already starting to become crippled with arthritis, although she tried to keep herself warm with memories of her home in Hungary, the vineyards, peach trees and sun-ripened melons. But on this evening the two hardly felt the cold as they talked and wept together, going over the same issues again and again. What if Api declared himself still unfit to serve, as he felt he was? What if he simply stayed and refused to return to the inferno? But then how could he support us in this tiny place when this terrible war, which they knew could not last much longer, was over? The few belongings and instruments they had left were in Berlin, and there Api was well known as an eye doctor and surgeon, so that he could rebuild his practice as soon as the war was over. The final argument which weighed heavily with him was that it was after all his duty as medical officer not to abandon his post at a time when he was most needed. However often they revisited their sad options, they came to the same terrifying conclusion: Api had to go back to Berlin. It was their life and their home, and it was his duty. They saw no other future. Nyussi, my mother and I would stay with farmer Ohlde in Suderburg. At least we were relatively safe.

Neither Api nor Nyussi got any sleep that night, and even I was restless sensing their unhappiness. They dreaded their separation and worried about the ever-more fragile and uncertain future. Although neither voiced it out loud, one question was always on their minds: would they ever see each other again? Lying awake and trying not to think of the morning, they turned their thoughts to their past happiness. They remembered fondly how they had played duets in their music room, or sat on their balcony unaware of the terror to come. Often that night they wept for their son who had fallen in Prague less than two months before. The next morning no one said much except to look forward to our reunion as soon as the war was over. We pictured how, immediately after the end, which could not be far off, Api would be on his way back to pick us up. Alone in Berlin, he often dwelled on that dreaded hour of parting, Tuesday 10 April at 5.15 p.m. precisely. He never forgot that day, the deathly sadness among us and the irony of the laughing spring day above.

A doctor acquaintance stopped at our cottage to take Api to Uelzen, from where he hoped to board a train back to Berlin. My grandmother quickly handed him a little parcel from our treasured supplies for the journey: a few *zwiebacks*, a piece of bread and, best of all, a little piece of *Speck* (the fatty bacon we liked to eat on dark bread). The *Speck* was a donation from the always generous Steinkes. Api took a last look at Nyussi, my mother and me standing in front of the timbered cottage, said a silent farewell to the peaceful Blue Mountain, and was gone. We would not hear from him again for many months. During that time Api often asked himself whether this was not the worst decision he had ever made in his life.

As soon as he had left us Api tried to relieve his anxiety by jotting down details of his journey back to Berlin on a torn-off piece of paper. Perhaps it was the beginning of a letter to us that would never be sent. The scrap nevertheless somehow found its way into my mother's lockbox. The trip was stressful for its endless delays and even more so for the torturous revolutions of his mind. He was lucky to find any trains at all that still functioned and when he climbed aboard the first one in Uelzen he was not surprised to see that it was filled to bursting. After only about 30 miles he had to change trains in Celle. At 6.30 p.m. he squeezed into the next overcrowded train, trying to get as close to a window as possible to catch a hint of fresh air. An hour later, just as the train pulled into Lehrte station near Hannover, the air-raid sirens sounded shrilly. Everyone rushed for shelter in the station bunker. While waiting, Api struck up a conversation with two air force lieutenants who were sitting on their rucksacks next to him. He told them that he planned to take the express train at 2.30 a.m. because it went directly to Berlin. The young men, however, advised him to leave Lehrte as fast as possible, even though he might not get far. After thirty minutes in the bunker they were told that there was to be no air raid after all. Back on the station platform, Api followed the advice of the lieutenants and waited for the 8.30 p.m. train which just went to Oebisfelde, 30 miles beyond Lehrte – but at least it was straight east in the direction of Berlin. While waiting he unwrapped and ate the provisions Nyussi had given him for the journey, keeping the *Speck* for later, and thought gratefully how she always took care of him, even to the point of depriving herself.

When he reached Oebisfelde he heard that the next train, which was due to arrive at 3.15 a.m., was eight to ten hours late. Perhaps, he thought, it would have been better to stay in the big Lehrte station after all. From here on out such doubts about any one of his decisions, big or small, would plague Api and drive him to distrust himself completely. At 4 a.m. he gave up on the express and took a slow train via Magdeburg. When they drew near to Magdeburg Api, like everyone else aboard, tried to avoid looking out, keeping his eyes turned away in order not to see the destruction beyond the windows. Nevertheless, he caught glimpses of heavy bomb damage. But for Api the most difficult part of that long and uncomfortable journey was the unrelenting stream of agonising thoughts from which he was unable to free himself. He kept asking himself the same questions: 'Should I have stayed in Suderburg after all? And what about my duty as a doctor and officer?' No doubt shaking his head, he wrote about his 'silly exaggerated sense of duty'. He knew that he could not act differently, that he had to return.

16

Russians at the Gates

If we step down the whole earth shall tremble!

For close to five years Api had known Berlin as a war zone, but just a few days after he returned, it became the front line. The city, which had continued to function through hundreds of air raids and years of carpet bombing, finally ground to a halt. Factories closed, streetcars stopped running, mail delivery and trash pickup ceased. The Russians, who had begun their march on Berlin on 16 April 1945, were at the gates.

Starting on Saturday 21 April 1945, Api wrote a detailed diary entry for each day, which he kept up until October, when he was finally able to leave Berlin. Each one is addressed to us and interwoven with prayers to help him through this time. The Russians were steadily coming closer to the centre and Api was fearfully gauging their progress by the sound of the shelling. In these last days of April, 40,000 tons of Russian artillery shells pounded the city. At the end one shell was exploding every five seconds in the government district, the so-called Citadel, where Api was.

On his return to Berlin, Api had tried to report back for duty but there was no one who could tell him where to go. So he went to work in the bunker on Albrechtstrasse near his former home where, in the cellar, was the auxiliary military clinic RL 104. Conditions were bad. They had light only for half an hour a day, and even then the Hindenburg lamps, made of tallow, threw only the dimmest rays. 'Again and again we had to make the old spent ones usable by reusing the fallen drops of tallow.' Nevertheless, Api kept reminding himself that it was a little better here than in the adjoining public shelter where hundreds of people were crowded together in the dark. Api was frustrated about how little could be done for the injured. There were far too many of them and many more had to be turned away altogether. He saw them outside in the rubble. Yet even the 'lucky' ones who were inside were lying on the bare and cold floor, whilst dust and chalk rained down on them from the ceiling as even the sturdy bunker was shaken by explosions. Toilets did not function and, without water or bandages, injuries had to stay largely untended. Groans and the whimpering of babies filled the air. Blood and grime ran down the surgeon's rubber apron. It smelled of excrement and old blood. Api saw no hope for anyone; he had only one wish: 'When – then I beg it only to be quick.'

The 21 April was a spring day of sunshine and showers in Berlin, although down in the cellar Api did not see much of it. I wonder whether he heard Goebbels' last 11 a.m. news conference from the Zoo Bunker in the nearby Tiergarten, in which Goebbels announced that he would stay in Berlin until victory. He added: '*Aber wenn wir abtreten, dann soll der Erdkreis erzittern!*', 'However, if we step down the whole earth shall tremble!' Meanwhile, Hitler hunkered down in his steel-reinforced bunker below the New Reich Chancellery. It was only a ten-minute walk from where Api was yet, of course, he knew nothing of what was happening there. Hitler was in a state of collapse, either raging or whimpering; sunk into himself, his left hand shaking uncontrollably, he shouted: 'Politics! I have nothing to do with politics any more. That just disgusts me.'

On the second day of his diary, 22 April, it had turned cold with a high barely reaching 7°C (45°F). Chilled and hungry after a sleepless night, Api went round the corner from Albrechtstrasse to see what was left of his former home on Luisenstrasse. In the distance he could hear long-range artillery fire, which meant the Russians were on their way. Although it was Sunday, stores had been ordered to stay open to distribute crisis rations of sausage, lentils, sugar and even a little coffee. Berliners jokingly called them suicide rations and no one was surprised that they did not materialise. Api checked the Pommer and Vorkastner stores where Nyussi used to shop and found one closed and the other besieged by hundreds of people. The shelves already were almost bare and he saw no hope of getting any food, so he continued on to his apartment building. He could no longer use the front stairs but the back stairs were navigable up to the second floor where his practice had been. The place smelled of smoke, dust and decay, but the ceiling appeared to have held, although there was no floor left above him.

As he surveyed the damage, a grenade hit the building next door at the same level where he was standing. The impact made him jump into the air, but he had a moment of hope nevertheless. It seemed to him that the attack had come from the west. That must be the Americans, he thought. It was the only hope left that the Americans would reach Berlin before the Russians. Little did he know that the Americans were not anywhere near Berlin. Already, on 28 March, General Eisenhower had reportedly told Field Marshal Montgomery to advance to the River Elbe and stop there. 'Berlin itself is no longer a particularly important objective,' he telegraphed in response to Montgomery's plea the day before for permission to lead a 'powerful and full-blooded thrust toward Berlin'.

From the moment he saw what had once been his surgery, Api cherished the hope that he could rebuild his practice. He could not live there yet, but whenever he felt any strength at all he returned to clean in order to get the place ready for patients and find a way to provide for us. Api left the apartment, still hungry but with some plans for the future. He decided to go across the street to the Charité, a walk he had taken so often in peacetime. Although the main buildings of the Charité had been heavily camouflaged, most of them had suffered considerable bomb damage. On his way he met a young colleague, Dr Heinz Kraaz, who had only recently finished his doctorate as a gynaecologist. He came to Api's rescue by inviting him to share his lunch.

During the next weeks and months they became fast friends. Heinz's visits always helped to shore up Api's failing energies. The young man did not have a wife and children to worry about and he also was possessed of an always positive, supportive and, even in this crisis, hopeful disposition. He helped Api at his most desperate times and the two enjoyed long, often philosophical evening talks, which, as Api noted frequently, were not political. Otherwise politics was what most people talked about, endlessly debating rumours and suppositions and fears. Although more than thirty years separated the two men, they had much in common. They shared a love for their profession, for helping people, a strong religious faith and a fundamentally conservative outlook. They also shared a joy of the heart. Although this was all but extinguished in my grandfather at this time, in Heinz's company he could even laugh sometimes.

That Sunday night, on 22 April, Api saw the east of Berlin in flames. 'Grenades roared through the blood red sky and fighter planes attacked even in the darkness.' He also heard a new noise: machine-gun fire coming from the east and the north, but very near. He reckoned that the Russians were as close as the *Schloss*, the royal palace, at the east end of Unter den Linden. Despite the noise he dropped off exhausted, for he had not slept for almost seventy hours.

When he was not at the Albrechtstrasse bunker, Api's other destination at that time was the university clinic at Ziegelstrasse 5–9, then RL 135. It was not far, just across the wide Friedrichstrasse and a little to the north, but it always took Api a long time to get there. He had to find his way over heaps of rubble, past abandoned tanks and streetcar rails stabbing the sky. Here and there one wall of a smouldering building was still standing and Api could see right inside a kitchen or a bedroom with its scorched furniture and torn wallpaper. It was like a doll's house wrecked by a giant. With bitter agreement he noticed a home-made poster attached to a shell of a house: *'Das danken wir dem Führer,'* 'For this we can thank the Führer.' In the last days of April he saw two officers hanging from a lamppost at the Friedrichstrasse station. Each had a bit of cardboard around his neck, on which was scribbled that all cowards would meet the same fate. Fanatical SS had executed the two for wearing civilian clothes under their uniforms.

The early morning of Wednesday 25 April, between 5.30 and 6.30 a.m., saw some of the heaviest bombardment of the inner city, burying the old paths Api knew through the ruins. Api, of course, was not aware that this attack had even reached Speer's monumental New Reich Chancellery. The ventilation system in Hitler's bunker had to be turned off since it no longer drew in fresh air but only sulphur and smoke.

He found the Ziegelstrasse clinic more than half destroyed by this attack, and all of it severely damaged. It had been a large complex consisting of two squares of red-brick buildings with two inner courtyards. As he walked along the wall of crumbling brick, Api noticed the sandstone half-relief of a Berlin bear just beside the entrance to one building. The bear has been the symbol of Berlin since the Middle Ages, and this one had remained intact although the city it represented was in ruins. When he entered the high hall, its floor covered ankle deep in dust and rubble, a fellow doctor met him to take him around. As they surveyed the damage, the doctor mentioned that the remaining headquarters of troop physicians might be moved to this location from their place on Jebenstrasse at the west end of the Tiergarten. Despite the heavy damage, this structure, long a part of the university clinics, had more resources and was a better place both for the wounded and the doctors than the bunker on Albrechtstrasse. Api hoped that he could work there.

The clinic was abuzz with rumours and also some eyewitness reports from people who had managed to come in from outer areas of Berlin. They said that the northern suburbs of Wittenau, Tegel and Reinickendorf had already been taken by the Russians. This meant that the Russians were all but in the centre of the city. They told Api that the first wave of attack was made up of Katyushas firing phosphorous rockets, which set everything aflame. The Germans called them *Stalinorgeln*, Stalin's organs, because going off they made a roaring sound like many organs playing. The Katyushas were followed by tanks which easily broke through any of the flimsy barricades. After the tanks came the infantry with grenades, sub-machine guns and rifles.

Then Api witnessed something which he had to report in his diary right away, perhaps to ease his mind a little: 'Just now chief medical officer 135 has buried 12 naked dead in a mass grave in Monbijou Park', the once beautiful park by the River Spree, aptly named 'My Treasure'. Monbijou Park was at the end of Ziegelstrasse, just across from the auxiliary clinic. Most parks in the city now served as burial sites and over the next days Api saw this scene repeated over and over in different locations. Despite what he had seen and heard at the Ziegelstrasse clinic, Api was disappointed when he was told that he could not stay there. It left him no other choice than to return to Albrechtstrasse. There, he noticed even further deterioration even though he had been gone only a few hours: 'We drank the last water that comes out of the heaters. Now people start to drink water from the River

Spree without being able to boil it. Then epidemics without hospitals, yes even without possibility of any quarters at all. Every child knows what happens then.' He went on to vent his impotent frustration at what he had seen on his way:

> One can hardly walk the streets. People die in the streets without there being any way of carrying them anywhere. Military clinics and hospitals have to reject everyone because of complete overcrowding, without water, without light. In some places I met up to 100 unattended heavy casualties with only two surgeons. Citizens are hungry and thirsty. Epidemics will not fail to come – a mass dying without any chance of improvement, an intoxication of the blood, a madness. Millions of furious people, in a powerless rage and despair, rebel against a brutality of tyrants which has never existed like this before, and they die helplessly!! Useless! An end, an end!! ... The situation is getting more horrible day by day. The cellars can no longer sustain the heavy bombardment. City power is gone completely so that we cannot recharge our emergency lighting. No quarters whatsoever, no bandages, and no food. Many soldiers are without food for three days. I fear *the very worst!* If there is no end, murder and manslaughter. Dead horses are cut up in the midst of bombardment, the meat eaten almost raw. No way of cooking, no water, no light! God take pity!!

The inner city was just about encircled by 2.5 million Russian soldiers. They had taken Tempelhof Airfield in the south-east and Spandau in the north-west. Alexanderplatz and Potsdamer Platz, both just a few minutes from Api's location, were under heavy attack and the once bombastic government buildings on Wilhelmstrasse already had been reduced to rubble. The whole inner city was smouldering from fires. Sulphurous yellow smoke hung heavy in the air and made it difficult to breathe. A violent thunderstorm on the morning of 26 April dampened everything but hardly cleared the air. At night Api was kept awake by heavy artillery fire and in the morning he confided to his diary: 'I don't know how I will get through this time. Despite a huge expense of energy, I can hardly work at all. I am constantly shaking with cold so that I can hardly write.'

On 26 April Api decided to make an attempt to reach the Command Centre Jebenstrasse. Perhaps there he would at last be given a proper assignment. The Command Centre, immediately across from the Zoo station, was a four-storey neo-classicist building of the early twentieth century that had served as an officers' mess of the Landwehr, the local militia, literally the 'defence of the country'. Now it also was the home of Major Pritsch's headquarters for the defence of Berlin.

It was an arduous and debilitating journey across the wasteland of the Tiergarten Api had so loved. The whole park was devastated with bomb craters and the trees were charred and broken, a nightmare landscape. The Command Centre was barely functioning. The formerly showy interior, once covered in colourful wall and ceiling paintings, lay in ruins. Many of the windows were broken and papers blew about in the draft. The chief physician, Dr Pellnitz, who was also an eye doctor, only advised Api to go back to Albrechtstrasse. Dr Pellnitz had no idea where he himself would go since the headquarters would soon be moved away from this dangerous area. Far from being able to help, he could tell Api only sad stories about fellow doctors who had committed suicide. When Api was back in the Albrechtstrasse bunker after this futile excursion, he was exhausted and assessed his own mental state at 'point zero'. He wrote: 'I have lost all confidence in myself and my initiatives. The conditions are horrible: no quarters in military hospitals and no transport of the sick ... Deplorable disorganization. Impossible to imagine. Impossible to describe.'

17

Abyss between Then and Now

… a wilderness of fire and dust, behind it, although already high in sky, the blood red moon.

In order to get a better idea about the places that appeared in the diary, Mike and I retraced Api's steps in June 2007. Of course, in the reunited Berlin, once again the booming capital of Germany, we were working under entirely different circumstances, crowded by tourists rather than soldiers and refugees, and bombarded with the noise of traffic instead of exploding artillery shells. Nevertheless, we found some reminders of the war, and saw places in the former East Berlin that still showed their wounds.

I had not been back to Berlin except for a brief visit in the late 1950s. Mike and I now stayed at a Westin Hotel at the intersection of Unter den Linden and Friedrichstrasse. Every step we took from there made us more aware of the abyss between then and now. We were strolling past fashionable stores while Api had made his laborious way through smoke and ruins, facing death at each step:

Towards evening the sky to the east is a ghastly sea of smoke. I creep out at 10 o'clock at night to the clinic under whistling grenades and bombs, a wilderness of fire and dust, behind it, although already high in sky, the blood red moon.

We began our tour at Luisenstrasse 41, no more than a ten-minute walk from the hotel. My mother had told me that it had been rebuilt exactly as it had been and was under historical landmark protection. Indeed, the stucco was freshly painted a pale yellow and the red tiles shone on the steep roof. I looked at the nameplates for the fourth floor. The only name listed was a social and religious discussion group. I found them in the telephone book and called to ask whether we could look at the apartment, explaining that from 1924 to 1945 my grandparents had lived there. Frau Bug, the woman in charge, readily agreed and we climbed up the sunlit stairwell to the fourth floor. Api must have gone up there a thousand times and I imagined my mother running down on her way to the streetcar and to school.

Frau Bug let us in and explained that the former apartment had been split into two, so what we saw was only one half of my grandparents' place. Then she allowed us to wander around on our own. The apartment was equipped with light and functional modern furniture so unlike what I had seen in pictures of my grandparents' time. Yet as we looked out the front windows we could see the cupola of the Reichstag, although the balcony they had enjoyed so much now belonged to the other apartment. The view from the back windows was even less changed. The windows gave out on to the first inner courtyard. Typical for Berlin apartment buildings, there are a series of such courtyards in the back which get successively smaller and darker. The front of the building used to be occupied by well-to-do professionals and the back by the poor and working class. In this way every building contained a mixture of social classes, living under very different circumstances but in close proximity. The first courtyard into which we were looking from the apartment was done in stucco painted yellow like the front of the building. The next two were exposed brick, as we discovered when we were again downstairs.

There was nothing more to see in this shiny new apartment, since even the layout was altered because of the divided space. After we had thanked Frau Bug for letting us in, we left to inspect the neighbourhood. Right across from the building I found the little triangular park my mother had told me about, the Karlplatz, which was just outside the gates to the

Charité. On a pedestal at its centre stood a bronze sculpture of Professor Rudolf Virchow (1821–1902), founder of the field of social medicine and known as the 'Father of Pathology'. The monument, which survived the Second World War, shows a man fighting a lion, perhaps to symbolise the great physician conquering the wild animal of disease. Luisenstrasse had been just east of the Berlin Wall under the jurisdiction of Communist East Germany. Now, over fifteen years after reunification, the area was becoming Westernised and gentrified. We noticed a wine bar and a tapas restaurant and I bought a wonderfully light and flaky almond horn, a *Mandelhörnchen*, one of my childhood favourite treats, in a bakery nearby. Most of the east side of Luisenstrasse where our apartment was had been filled in with new buildings, but on the western side of the street we still saw quite a few weed-grown and empty lots.

Next we went in search of my mother's elementary school. I knew that it was located on Albrechtstrasse, which runs one block east of Luisenstrasse. It is a short street. At the south side it ends at Friedrichstrasse station and to the north it runs into Schumannstrasse near the Deutsches Theatre. I did not know the house number, but remember my mother telling me that her school was an older structure nestled among taller apartment buildings. We began at the station, walking north and scanning both sides of the street for a small house. And there it was, on the east side of the street, a small narrow structure of yellow brick squeezed in between larger ones. It somehow had survived that onslaught of rebuilding during the *Gründerzeit*, the founder's period at the turn of the nineteenth century when Berlin blossomed into a world city.

After taking pictures, we walked further up the street not looking for anything in particular. Suddenly at the corner of Albrechtstrasse and Reinhardtstrasse a massive grey block of reinforced concrete, five stories high with rows of slit openings, loomed in front of us. It sat there, huge and somewhat sinister, looking so completely out of place among the apartment buildings, coffee shops and bakeries that lined the street. It seemed like a dinosaur from a different age. In a moment of excited recognition I exclaimed to Mike: 'Look, this must be the bunker Api had written so much about. I had never expected to see it.' Looking at it more closely we noticed that the bunker had been converted into a museum of contemporary art and that a penthouse with a roof garden had also been added. We could see some greenery peeking out at the top, although this did little to soften its aspect. Having actually seen the bunker helped me to visualise Api's descriptions, and its somehow threatening aspect in the midst of today's apartments and shops brought me closer to his time.

After the discovery of the bunker, Mike and I crossed Friedrichstrasse and turned into Ziegelstrasse. On our way to the former clinic, we got perhaps just a hint of what it must have been like in 1945. Here the war was still leaving its traces, just as it was on me and my project. Although only a few blocks north of elegant and bustling Unter den Linden, the street we encountered was shabby and deserted. On the south side it was flanked by the old brick buildings of the university that stretch for almost its whole length, and we spotted the Berlin bear Api had described at a corner. On the north side we saw nothing but broken-down structures, still showing the bullet holes of over half a century ago. In between gaped empty spaces where once had stood buildings. Now there were only rubbish and weeds. Altogether the street gave a dilapidated, abandoned impression and showed us how long it takes for the scars of war to heal over.

In the afternoon Mike and I followed Api's journey from Albrechtstrasse to Jebenstrasse, but under much happier circumstances. Before we set out across the park, we enjoyed a glass of wine at the lavishly refurbished Hotel Adlon at Pariser Platz 1, next to the Brandenburg Gate on the south side of Unter den Linden. Sipping our wine by the marble fountain, we talked about the Adlon's illustrious history. Before the war it had been the favourite meeting place for journalists, diplomats, film stars and fashionable ladies out on a *Linden Bummel*, a Linden promenade. At the end of the war the Adlon was the last of Berlin's grand hotels left standing, serving as a refuge for the sick and wounded. The barber shop in the basement had been hastily fitted out as an operating room, and the dead were stacked in the once beautiful Goethe garden at the rear. At the end of April the hotel had opened its famed 250,000-bottle wine cellar to the public. Waiters in their dusty tuxes served wine and champagne, gingerly stepping over debris and shards from the chandeliers. Although heavily damaged, the Adlon survived the war but, on 3 May 1945, the grand building finally collapsed as it was consumed by fire.

Sitting in luxury, it was hard for us to picture the desolation Api had seen here. We left the Adlon and stepped out on to Pariser Platz, where we were met by a bustle of tourists taking pictures of the Brandenburg Gate. My mind wandered to the thousands that had stood there in 1914, cheering and sticking flowers in the gun barrels of young soldiers, as indeed Api must have done. Less than twenty years later the square was filled with brown-shirted SA storm troopers carrying torches and chanting the *Horst Wessel* song to celebrate Hitler becoming chancellor. Then at the time of the diary the square was taken up by dead and wounded soldiers.

From the Brandenburg Gate we set out across the Tiergarten. It was a cool but sunny afternoon and we enjoyed the lovely hike through tree-shaded paths, much like Api and Nyussi had done before the war. But when we got to Jebenstrasse, I felt once again a little closer to Api's experience. At first I almost did not want to go down that empty and narrow street bounded on one side by the Zoo station wall. There were a group of men and women gathered halfway down, perhaps waiting for a soup kitchen to open. The grey, official-looking buildings on the other side still had a pre-war era about them, even though they had been renovated. We found the former Command Centre, which now was a museum of photography. It had been restored just three years earlier, in 2004. When we stepped inside, we saw no more traces of what Api had found. Even the showy ball room, the *Kaiser Saal*, or Emperor's Hall, had been restored to its former splendour. It brought home to us the impossibility of bridging the abyss between then and now.

18

Blocked on All Sides

All of Berlin a field of ruins more so than after the heaviest bombardment. Streets full of holes and rubble. Hardly navigable, wires, trees and such a dust that one can hardly keep one's eyes open. All the bridges are barricaded.

Although hopeless and worn out after his futile journey to Jebenstrasse, Api was too anxious just to stay at the Albrechtstrasse bunker. He felt that somehow he had to obtain a definite assignment, preferably at an eye clinic, 'where I could do some good even in my condition'. All day he worried about this until, at 8 p.m., he rushed out in search of the chief physician. Under heavy bombardment he had to duck from cover to cover to make his way, otherwise the streets were deserted. He reached his destination (which he did not specify in the diary) but was told that the chief physician was gone. To his great surprise, however, someone else authorised his move to the eye station of the Auxiliary Military Clinic RL 112 in Wilmersdorf, the very one he had been trying to reach a few days before. Even a car and driver would be standing ready at 4 a.m. to take him to Wilmersdorf and, incredibly to him, he was offered another option, which had been denied just the previous day. He was now given permission to work at Ziegelstrasse RL 135 under Professor Löhlein.

Api may have known the professor from before the war, since he had been in charge of the eye clinic at Ziegelstrasse, which was connected to the Charité. They were almost the same age. Professor Löhlein was born in 1882 in Berlin, the son of a professor of gynaecology. He was a tall man who wore his hair very short and parted on one side, as did Api. He had a high forehead, a thick white moustache and penetrating blue eyes. I have read that Professor Löhlein had been Hitler's personal ophthalmologist. Ever since his eye injury in 1918, Hitler feared for his sight and needed the reassurance of the specialist. If Api was aware of Professor Löhlein's role, he did not mention it in his diary.

Suddenly Api had not one but two possibilities, and it threw him into a new consternation. Not trusting his decisions, he did not know what to do:

> Well, now again a conflict: the 112 eye station already lies within the *HKL* [*Hauptkampflinie*: main battle line] and will therefore be run over earlier. If I connect with Ziegelstrasse I can stay in my relatively safe cellar for the time being, won't have the dangerous commute and can remain close to my apartment and my instruments.

At 10 p.m. Api decided to venture out once more 'under whistling grenades' on his way to Ziegelstrasse to make doubly sure that they would have him there.

He reached the clinic unhurt and it was confirmed that he could work there now. Nevertheless, on his way back he kept thinking about his options and could not make up his mind. 'At the last minute I decide to stay and go to military hospital Ziegelstrasse. Give God that for once I should have chosen correctly, even just because of you whom I love above all, above all. God be with you!!' Although he had finally decided on Ziegelstrasse, he was unable to stick with his choice. Terror and exhaustion had enervated him and taken away any initiative. As soon as he had opted for one solution, his lack of self-confidence led him to reverse himself. This back-and-forth process served as only further proof that he was right in doubting himself. He was correct, however, about Wilmersdorf already being in the main battle zone. It was in fact taken by the Red Army just two days later, on 28 April. Therefore, Api made up his mind once and for all to stick with his plan to stay at Ziegelstrasse and work with Professor Löhlein.

Despite having just resolved this, Api continued to plague himself for the rest of the night with where to go, which place to choose. Just before finally dropping into a weary sleep, he reassured himself that it was the right decision to stick with the Ziegelstrasse option. 'I am a terrible fellow, torturesome indecision impersonated.' But he did not sleep long and finally got up before 4 a.m. on Friday 27 April and once again reversed his decision:

> At 4 in the morning I again had doubts what to do. I am running until the last minute between driving and staying. Remain undecided back and forth. Finally I drive after all. Artillery bombardment small. But all of Berlin a field of ruins more so than after the heaviest bombardment. Streets full of holes and rubble. Hardly navigable, wires, trees and such a dust that one can hardly keep one's eyes open. All the bridges are barricaded.

Blocked on all sides, Api and the driver decided to motor straight across the paths of the Tiergarten where, ironically, the tall Victory Column was one of the few structures still standing. It commemorated German war victories as well as the unification of Germany under Bismarck. Since 1941 the column had been camouflaged with netting and the winged golden goddess on top, whom Berliners liked to call Golden Elsa, was covered with brown paint. All around the monument burnt-out tanks were abandoned and the dead lay unburied. Trying not to look too closely at what surrounded them, they made it to the other end of the Tiergarten, to the big square then called the Knie, which Api remembered had been created in 1902 as the western end station of the first underground. Today the square has been renamed Ernst Reuter Platz.

At the Knie they came under low-level attack from Russian planes, the 'sewing machines' strafing the city. When it was over, they drove on and finally reached Command Centre Jebenstrasse by the Zoo station. It had taken the driver almost three hours to cover a stretch of about 2 miles. Api found Dr Pellnitz, who still held out there although he had lost contact with his clinics. The planned relocation of the medical department obviously had not occurred, probably because there was no one to organise it and no place to go. Dr Pellnitz showed Api the latest copy of the *Panzerbär* (the *Tank Bear*) 'Combat Paper for the Defenders of Greater Berlin'. Its cover always displayed a bear holding a *Panzerfaust* in each paw. This means literally a 'tank fist', which was a small anti-tank weapon even the children and old men of the *Volkssturm* (the People's Militia) called up at the eleventh hour could hold in their hands. Despite all evidence to the contrary, the 27 April copy carried the headline: 'Bulwark against Bolshevism. Berlin: Mass Grave for Soviet Tanks.' Both Api and Dr Pellnitz could only shake their heads in disbelief.

Soon after leaving the Command Centre, on their way to Wilmersdorf, it became clear to both Api and the driver that they could no more reach their goal by car than Api had been able to on foot earlier: 'Impossible to get there. All the streets buried under rubble; the enemy at the Circle Line Wilmersdorf. Caught in the midst of battling troops, we are sent back.' At this point the driver left, but Api did not say anything about the man's plans.

Now what to do? Return to the Zoo and go back to the decision he had made yesterday? Or stay just north of where he had got stuck and report to the military clinic RL 151 on Nikolsburger Platz?

Since from Zoo to Friedrichstrasse only a footmarch is possible, I stay. Pellnitz refers me to 151. Dr Siebert, chief medical officer 151, says yes. But because of an absolute lack of space he wants to house me on the second totally evacuated storey, and then once again a heavy high calibre bombardment gets under way.

During a lull in the bombardment, Api inspected the place:

The corridors and the middle hall are for untended wounded; 14 corpses wrapped in oil paper are dropped in the park, a little earth on top!! No water. The stink of toilets. Unusable. If only I could get back!! An opportunity to drive is out of the question. Against urgent warnings, I decide on a foot march.

Api set out from the devastated Nikolsburger Platz filled with misgivings. He felt that he had to get away from that misery, even though nothing much better awaited him on the other end. Heading east toward Kurfürstendamm, he crossed the once broad Hohenzollerndamm trying not to look at the hills of rubble on either side which narrowed the street to a lane. He made his way into Fasanenstrasse, which had lost most of its trees. When he reached Pariserstrasse only a couple of blocks from his starting point the trouble began. He later recorded it all in a breathless and simple language unusual for him:

> Already in Pariser Strasse increasing bombardment with high calibre weapons. At Rankeplatz I thought my last hour had come! Two heavy ones 50 meters to my right. I try to run across the square, two heavy hits 50 meters in front of me. Houses only ruins. I crouch, together with a *Volkssturm* guy, behind a suburban fence. Again 4 heavy ones right near us. I must try to move forward into Rankestrasse. After 30 paces, two of the heaviest 100 paces ahead of me. When I turn back into Joachimstalerstrasse, again 2 heavy ones 70 meters ahead. Three cars of a parked convoy in high flames.

Then, he spotted a small car with two officers and a woman:

> I immediately cross the street, force them to stop, and jump in. Straight through the sea of flames – my brows singed – without sight for 50 meters straight ahead. When we are out, again two pot hits on the old spot. Car drives across Friedrichstrasse. I knew the only usable path and got through, uttering the most heartfelt prayers while grenades continually exploded.

Api's path across the ruins may well have been the same – or one much like it – that was taken a few days later by the last people to flee Hitler's bunker on 1 May. That night, at 11 p.m., Hitler's private secretary, the short-legged fat Martin Bormann, Brigade Commander Mohnke, Hitler's bodyguard, his dietitian Constanze Manzialy, his young secretary Traudl Junge and others were attempting a last-minute break out of Berlin. The first thing they saw after they left Hitler's bunker was the bloody horror of the emergency clinic under the old Reich Chancellery where doctors sawed off legs and arms without anaesthesia, and the dead and wounded lay about in mangled heaps together with scattered body parts. Next they crawled through pitch-black subway tunnels toward Friedrichstrasse station, their feet often slipping on something soft: a person either dead or unconscious. But they moved on, hoping not to lose the other members of their group in the darkness. They avoided crossing the River Spree at the heavily guarded Weidendammer Bridge, one of the main ways out of the city. Instead they crept around Friedrichstrasse to Ziegelstrasse and from there to the Charité.

One member of that group was Ernst-Günther Schenck, who had served as a doctor in the Reich Chancellery. He described how, sweating and bruised, they inched their way through that labyrinth in the ruins:

> The path which we now entered was completely hidden and had obviously been forged by pioneers through an entire district ... It used old courtyards, cellars, parts of demolished apartments, darted sideways around larger ruins, ran along a small street, and wound its way up and down over rubble and crumbled walls. The path looked lost and yet could not be missed.

The location Schenck describes tallies exactly with where Api was going on his return from Nikolsburger Platz. So it may well have been the same labyrinthine path through a no-man's-land that took Api back to the Albrechtstrasse cellar. When he finally collapsed in his cellar on that Friday, 27 April, it felt almost like home: 'Arrival!! ... Luckily a few old peeled potatoes. Potatoes, dry bread, no water!'

19

Wrapped Up in the Flag

Einigkeit und Recht und Freiheit

When we returned to Berlin in June 2008, Mike and I also visited Nikolsburger Platz in the district of Berlin-Charlottenburg. On our way there, we went along the tree-lined side streets west of Kurfürstendamm, which once again had uninterrupted strings of beautiful apartment buildings, some old and some new or rebuilt. It was an up-scale neighbourhood, away from traffic yet close to the centre. Mike read the menus at the many inviting restaurants and wanted to try each one. I admired the patisseries in the bakery displays and the fine food in the grocery stores, wishing we could have just one such deli in South Bend. However, on this day of 29 June 2008 the usually quiet streets were packed with young people. Around the open-air tables of corner bars the crowds were particularly thick and noisy. Many wore big fuzzy hats and had their faces painted in the black, red and gold of the German flag. We learned that this was the day of the final of the UEFA European Football Championship between Germany and Spain. Although the game was played in Vienna and started at eight at night, by four in the afternoon 500,000 fans had gathered by the Brandenburg Gate and the square had to be closed. The lucky ones who had got in waited for hours to watch the game on a giant TV screen and cheer for their team. We stayed well away from that area. But Mike said how much better it was to have the Brandenburg Gate besieged by football fans instead of storm troopers or even the cheering crowds and the soldiers of the summer of 1914.

Yet as we walked toward Nikolsburger Platz, I felt perturbed by all the German flags I saw. They were everywhere I looked: on cars, on buildings, in restaurants. Everyone who strolled along the streets carried at least one flag, waving it in the air or even wrapped up in it. It made me feel very uncomfortable to walk among all the black, red and gold. My generation had been taught to avoid the flag. It was seen as a sign of a dangerous nationalism which had led to the Nazi terror. My school had no German flag anywhere and when we gathered for ceremonial celebrations, such as the beginning of the school year or even graduation, the national anthem had no part in it. Instead we sang the *Ode to Joy* from the end of Beethoven's *Ninth Symphony*, which contains the lines 'All men become brothers where your soft wing dwells'. Today the *Ode to Joy* serves as the anthem for the EU. While I lived in Germany until the early 1960s I did not once hear or sing the German national anthem, and to this day I do not like to be surrounded by flag-waving people, of any nation. I imagine that others of my generation also will not lose their anxiety about seeing a sea of flags, but especially German flags.

Weeks later I talked to a younger German acquaintance, I think she was in her forties. In the course of our conversation I happened to mention my unease about seeing Berlin blanketed in German flags. To my surprise she responded that, on the contrary, she thought it was healthy that Germans now could wave their flags like other nations without feeling troubled about the past: 'We cannot always live in the shadow of Hitler.' I had never thought of it in that way and can appreciate its value for a new Germany. Perhaps it signifies a sort of liberation, another step away from the Nazi period. I admit that this is a new and reassuring view, but that does not mean I can overcome my discomfort at a profuse display of any flag.

I also believe that some of my concern still clings to Germany altogether, and our national anthem is an indication of this. The old national anthem, the one that dates back to the revolution of 1848 and was adopted by the Weimar Republic, has been reinstated. It is now sung on festive occasions in Germany, but only the third stanza has been designated as the legal anthem.

It begins with '*Einigkeit und Recht und Freiheit*', that is, 'Unity, and Law, and Freedom'. The first stanza, the infamous and misunderstood '*Deutschland über alles*', is not allowed to be sung. In fact, it has become illegal in Germany to voice it. However, as it was used by the revolutionaries of 1848, the '*über alles*' did not mean that Germany should rule above all. It rather meant that a unified Germany should be the goal above all else, for only then could there be law and freedom for all. Germany at the time was split up into many countries, duchies and even kingdoms, each with its own feudal laws which were to guarantee the continued domination of the ruling class. But today few people remember the idealistic and revolutionary significance of this '*über alles*'. Our view is blocked by Hitler's insane attempt to impose himself on the world and, indeed, set up Germany '*über alles*'. So those words seem to have lost forever their original intent and have become tainted with the horror and bloodshed of the Nazi years.

When we finally reached Nikolsburger Platz all was quiet since there were no bars or outdoor restaurants there. Bright green grass grew in the centre of the square with a pretty border of red and yellow flowers. The apartment buildings that circled around it were new, each with tall windows and balconies, framed by linden trees. Then on the north side of the square we spotted one large, older building of stucco and brick. It was a school. This must have been the place which had housed RL 151 at the end of the war. Just then an old woman was laboriously walking along the park. I approached her gingerly and told her about Api. When she seemed comfortable to talk to me, I asked her whether she had been here in 1945. She said that she had and then she confirmed that the school had served as a makeshift hospital. The only other survivor of the war in this square was a 1ft-high iron rail with little decorated posts that marked off the green space. Everything else must have been reduced to rubble when Api was there.

That night in our hotel we were kept awake by shouting and firecrackers. Germany had lost the game 0–1, but that did not stop the crowds from parading up and down Kurfürstendamm, laughing and singing, and, no doubt, waving their flags.

20

Mood Reports

The end of the war or my own! If only one could
lead the Executioner of Berlin through this misery.

A t the end of April the Russians were coming ever closer and
the shooting was almost uninterrupted as three Soviet armies
concentrated their attack on the city centre. Marshal Zhukov's
troops fired from the Landwehr Canal immediately south of the
Citadel. Stalin had given Zhukov, the liberator of Stalingrad, the honour of
being the first to capture Berlin. General Bersarin, who soon was to become
the popular Commandant of Berlin, was stationed at Alexanderplatz to the
east and Marshal Konev's troops were at Wilmersdorf, south-west of the
centre, the very area Api had tried to reach. Against this overwhelming
force stood only scattered remnants of German units, some SS and the
ragtag *Volkssturm* with their *Panzerfausts*. Yet many of them, especially the
Waffen-SS, refused to give up and carried on guerrilla warfare against the
Russians, which cost both sides untold lives.

The Albrechtstrasse bunker, although still standing solidly, shook as it
had with the bombs. Api feared that neither the cellar nor his mind could
withstand this onslaught much longer:

Gradually one collapses psychically. If only I were properly at a military hospital and – an end. The end of the war or my own! If only one could lead the Executioner of Berlin through this misery. If they haven't turned insane from their bestiality, if they still believe in any kind of personal responsibility, if their often praised love of the people has even a glimmer of genuineness, their decision would not be in doubt, even if they would have to give themselves up. That they cannot prevent anyhow.

It was Saturday night, 28 April, when Api railed against the Nazis in his diary and wished for the end of the war or his own. That same night, not far away, Hitler married Eva Braun in their bunker 25m below ground. She wore her high-necked black taffeta dress, which was his favourite, and everyone in the bunker feverishly drank champagne and ate caviar sandwiches into the early morning. The air was sticky and oppressive and plaster rained down on the drunken celebrants. It covered their champagne and the silver trays of salmon, lobster and goose-liver pâté in a thin layer of dust. Shortly after the ceremony Hitler retired. He spent the rest of the night writing his political testament in which he denied that he had started the war and instead blamed a conspiracy of international Jewish leaders for the disaster.

Even in this hopeless situation when they knew defeat was inevitable, the Nazi organisation and the military maintained what they called a *Mundpropagandaaktion*, a propaganda machinery by word of mouth. It was to create trust in the leaders and strengthen the conviction that the war had to be won. Military men who were injured or otherwise unable to fight were assigned to mingle with the population, dressed in civilian clothes, and spread whatever the slogan of the day stipulated. After an air raid they took positions at bunkers and tried to pacify those who were desperate or help old ladies reach their homes, all the while doing their 'propaganda by word of mouth' about a rescue of Berlin. General Walther Wenck's relief army would, they promised, run down the enemy and save Berlin. This message was also spread by the *Panzerbär*, which until its last issue on 29 April, kept talking about the strength of Wenck's relief army and its tank units. On 22 April the headline had quoted Hitler: 'Berlin Stays German!'

Similar posters of '*BERLIN BLEIBT DEUTSCH*' had been stuck on the ruins of buildings and on any lampposts still standing. In addition, Goebbels' propaganda machinery put out this flier:

> *Berliner! Haltet aus, die Armee Wenck ist zum Entsatz angetreten, nur noch wenige Tage und Berlin ist wieder frei.*

> Berliners! Bear up, the Wenck army is coming to your rescue, only a few more days and Berlin will be free again!

Goebbels went on to order the population to fight for every street, every house and every ruin, to fight to the last man and the last cartridge. Women were urged to take up the defence of their city and step into the place of fallen *Volkssturm* men and boys.

Although Berliners did not believe that General Wenck would come to their aid, some of this 'word of mouth propaganda' may have helped, for makeshift signs appeared on destroyed buildings proclaiming: 'Our walls are breaking but not our hearts.' Perhaps, however, such sentiments were simply a sign of how unproductive it was to bomb civilians. In London after the Blitz a popular poem expressed exactly the same sentiment, in the same words even. Greta Brigg's *London Under Bombardment* has these lines:

> *The bombs have shattered my churches,*
> *Have torn my streets apart.*
> *But they have not bent my spirit*
> *And they shall not break my heart.*

In addition to spreading hope in the face of certain defeat, the propaganda men had another job. They were instructed to engage in an elaborate participant observation all across Berlin and then report back on the mood of the population. In contrast to the propaganda they had been ordered to disseminate, these reports were truthful and specific. The observers took down, word for word, conversations they had overheard while standing in line at stores, cinemas, sitting in pubs or waiting in stations. As early as 13 February 1945 one of the observers reported a remark in, of all places, the Kaffee Alois on Wittenberg Square near the Kurfürstendamm. The coffee house belonged to Hitler's half-brother Alois and was a favourite spot for storm troopers. A guest told his partner: 'The situation looks bad. I have already destroyed my copy of *Mein Kampf* and Hitler's picture.'

These detailed *Stimmungsberichte*, or mood reports, give a fascinating picture of daily life under the bombs. Even when faced with the threat of death and disintegration people worried about the ordinary details of everyday life. The reporters heard the understandable concerns about food, coal for heating and the conditions in bunkers, but people also expressed their annoyance at dirt in stations, at noisy waiters during official military reports, at impolite railway employees and at street lamps that were left burning by day wasting electricity. I wonder whether this was a typical reaction of people trying to maintain a sense of normalcy amidst chaos, or whether this showed a characteristically German fussiness?

At the end of April the defence of the inner city rested on three flak towers that were to protect the government centre, the Citadel: Humboldthain in the north, Friedrichshain in the east and Zoo in the west. The towers were built of 8ft of steel-reinforced concrete, six stories high. They could not be blown up even after the war. The flak towers had their own water, electricity and food, and even their own hospitals with operating theatres. The Zoo tower alone sheltered as many as 30,000 people and, since it was closest to Hitler's bunker, it also served as Goebbels' headquarters.

On 29 April, a Sunday, all telephone communication between Berlin and the outside world was broken. The city and its remaining 2.5 million people were completely cut off. Berlin had become a no-man's-land for the invasion of the Red Army. Russians had put an even narrower noose around the Citadel – north at Weidendammer Bridge, east at Lustgarten, south at Potsdamer Platz and west at Tiergarten – and only a few hundred metres separated them from the New Reich Chancellery. Historian Antony Beevor gives this haunting description of the night of 29/30 April:

In the centre of Berlin that night the flames in bombarded buildings cast strange shadows and a red glow on the otherwise dark streets. The soot and dust in the air made it almost unbreathable. From time to time there was the thunder of masonry collapsing. And to add to this terrifying effect, searchlight beams moved around above, searching a night sky in which the Luftwaffe had ceased to exist.

Without any news – even Goebbels' leaflets had finally ceased – Api could rely only on his immediate senses; what he saw and heard around him. He heard infantry fire nearby and machine-gun fire, which sounded as if it came from the direction of the Weidendammer Bridge at Friedrichstrasse, and he saw a number of disabled tanks on Wilhelmstrasse:

> The enemy's artillery is becoming more oppressive every day and we use 3–4 Flak [short for *Fliegerabwehrkanonen*, anti-aircraft guns] against, in my estimation, 100 who are firing in our district alone. There is no telephone or other means of communication with other battle units. A situation report for our district – even our remaining military command knows nothing of the others!! – is only issued on the basis of presumed eye witness reports. One can hardly step into the street. Beautiful artillery is standing useless in the Tiergarten because of lack of gas.

Api felt totally alone, isolated and hopeless. Although he worked in the medical cellar, he had not been able to establish a connection to any post or team of doctors. Thus he was not only cut off from us but even from his job as military doctor, which had been the main reason he had returned to Berlin in the first place. He did what he could to help the sick and injured, but it all seemed so senseless. He relieved his anger and frustration in berating those responsible for all this misery:

> Never before have there been such sadistic heartlessly brutal tyrants ... I am mentally and emotionally completely at an end, broken by the inexpressible mental and bodily misery which irresponsible people, without sense or purpose, have brought to over two and a half million desperate citizens. They better watch out!

As always in his most desperate moments, Api opened his diary, took out the little pencil that was attached to it by a loop at the front and began to talk with us: 'This morning at 8am,' he wrote late on 29 April, 'I had the distinct feeling that you, my world, were very close to me.' In his thoughts he looked out of the little cottage window with us and saw the peaceful landscape with the Blue Mountain in the distance. What a difference that scene offered him compared to what he saw all around. He forced himself to visualise it for as long as possible as a means of calming his nerves.

Reality, however, intruded all too soon:

Just now I have been looking for spaces where one can at least have the sick sit down or lay them on the ground for the night, without doors or windows, but at least protected from rain and safe from grenade splinters, although cold without padding. Corpses lie in a chapel of the Ziegelstrasse Clinic, for the most part without clothes, men and women together in layers! The streets are rubble fields that are hardly passable. Just now again a huge drum fire; women and girls cry desperately! It cannot be imagined or described what tortures these poor people who are more or less condemned to death have to suffer at the thought of perishing somewhere under the open sky without care, the victims of hunger revolts, themselves famished, and then fall into the hands of the Russians. I hope and pray that you have no idea of our situation. For even after the fall of Berlin the hunger monster will be terrible and it will be more horrible with each day of delay. Therefore, despite everything, I wish the end!!

21

Humans are Fiercer

Twenty-three soldiers one after the other. I had to be
stitched up in hospital. I never want to have anything
to do with any man again.

A t 10.50 p.m. on Monday 29 April Marshal Zhukov's troops
raised the hammer-and-sickle flag on the crumbling Reichstag.
Stalin had kept his promise and allowed the much-decorated
'Victory Marshal', and not his rival Marshal Konev, to be the
first to reach the Reichstag. Ironically, the building which once had housed
the German Parliament had not been in use since 1933, when part of it was
burnt down. From his apartment window Api must have seen the flames
shooting up from the Reichstag on 27 February 1933. Hitler had accused
the communists of arson and solidified his position as the man to create
order and fight international communism. I wonder whether in 1945 Api
noticed the Reichstag in flames once again, this time from Russian artillery.
The Third Reich had begun, and now it was ended with the burning
Reichstag.

The attack on Berlin had cost the Russians 70,000 men in house-to-
house fighting among the ruins, and even now SS troops continued to
attack from the basement of the smouldering Reichstag. According
to Russian statistics, the entire Russian losses of Operation Berlin were
304,887 men.

Journalist Vasily Grossmann described what was happening just a few blocks from where Api was. Although Grossmann had gone through the terror that was Stalingrad – one of the bloodiest battles in the history of warfare – he was overwhelmed by conditions in Berlin, the wasteland of smoking ruins, the mountains of dead, the refugees and prisoners of war. Grossmann walked around in a state of shock. When he came to the Zoo in the Tiergarten he struck up a conversation with the primate keeper. The gorilla, supposedly the largest in Europe, lay dead in her cage, as were most of the other animals. Fighting around the Zoo flak tower had been particularly heavy. Grossmann asked the primate keeper, who had looked after the ape for thirty-seven years:

'Was she fierce?'

'No,' he replied, 'she just roared loudly. Humans are much fiercer.'

Grossmann also watched the Red Army celebrate their long-fought-for victory. Api mentioned nothing of these celebrations in the heart of Berlin, perhaps because he spent his time in the bunker cellar. But according to Grossmann, 'the tanks are so covered in flowers and red banners that you can hardly see them ... Everyone is dancing, singing, laughing. Hundreds of coloured signal flares are fired into the air. Everyone salutes the victory with bursts from sub-machine guns, rifles, and pistols.' On Pariser Platz by the Brandenburg Gate, right in front of the Hotel Adlon, Soviet soldiers roasted an ox for the celebration, shouting gleefully: '*Krieg kaput! Hitler kaput!*'

Although Berliners had longed for an end to the war, they were deathly afraid of the Russians. Refugees from the East had come with horrific tales of murder and rape. To calm the population's fears, the Soviets dropped leaflets saying, 'The Red Army comes to you as Liberators'. But people could not believe that and they were proved right to be wary. The Russians had suffered so much and for so long from this enemy that they at last had conquered; when they were finally in control of Berlin, they went on a rampage of rape and looting which terrified Berliners no less than the bombing had done. Seen from the Russians' impoverished state everyone in Berlin was a capitalist, what with their watches, radios, carpets and toilets. '*Uri, Uri,*' they shouted in their version of the German word *Uhr*, meaning watch. Soon their arms were covered in watches all the way above their elbows. Wherever they spotted a bottle of liquor, they drank it. And when there was no *Schnapps*, they made do with pure alcohol and even tried the German cologne called *Kölnisch Wasser*. The promise of the Russians as liberators was further undermined when they proceeded to arrest any German in a uniform, even firemen or railway workers. Long lines of grey-faced and ragged prisoners of war were marched through the streets of Berlin on their way East.

At night, when the soldiers were drunk, they terrorised women. An estimated 100,000 women were raped in Berlin during the early days of the occupation. Women blackened their faces with coal and dirt; they dressed in rags; they did everything they could to make themselves look old and ugly, but nothing worked. They were unable to lock themselves away in the ruins in which they lived, and the Russians broke in on them wherever they tried to conceal themselves. Even nurses in hospitals did not escape the attacks of Russian soldiers, who checked the beds of the sick to make sure no nurse was hiding under the covers. Ursula von Kardoff, a journalist who worked as editor for the culture section of the *Deutsche Allgemeine Zeitung* in Berlin, recorded in her diary what a young woman told her. Her experience was by no means unique at that time: 'Twenty-three soldiers one after the other. I had to be stitched up in hospital. I never want to have anything to do with any man again.'

Among all the nightmarish experiences Api recorded, he never once mentioned the rapes. I can only speculate about the reasons for this omission. He either thought this too horrible to share with us or, although it seems less likely, he had no immediate personal knowledge of rape.

22

You Not Lie

The Führer has died at the head of the courageous
defenders of the Reich capital.

Berlin had fallen but the fighting continued. As Api made his way
back and forth between Albrechtstrasse and Ziegelstrasse, he still
saw plenty of violence. On Tuesday 1 May he wrote hastily in
his diary, often crossing out lines because he was too exhausted
to find the right words: 'Toward 1.30 a.m. terrible carpet bombing. Our
quarter is burning on all sides and at all ends. Nowhere are the streets
passable because of rubble, smoke, and flames. We are imprisoned
by the fire.' A little later he added more extensively, voicing his anger
and frustration:

> our entire area is burning, Friedrichstrasse to Oranienburger Tor,
> Johannisstrasse, Ziegelstrasse, Artelleriestrasse to Oranienburger-
> strasse, and not a drop of water ... And the executioners in their
> bunkers [as he called the Nazi leadership], criminals!! Rome, Milano,
> and other foreign cities were given up to spare them, and they allow
> their own people to perish like dogs with hunger and fire and fratricide.
> The houses already are looted by civilians or tramps. Several times
> a day we have to destroy weapons and munitions, which our own

troops drop off by our building, since we have no communication with any department.

Api is referring to one of the first orders put out by the Russian occupation that all weapons had to be turned in immediately. Api even gave up his old ornamental sword from the First World War. I have seen pictures of it from the 1920s when Api was wearing his dress uniform.

That afternoon, on his way to Ziegelstrasse, Api was hit by a grenade splinter. Fortunately it merely grazed his hip. It was only a light injury, soon forgotten on his journey into a nightmare world. Around Friedrichstrasse dead and dying soldiers had collapsed on the ground, tanks driving over their bodies. Looking south toward the Weidendammer Bridge across the River Spree, Api saw Russian tanks blocking the road. This bridge, which the last people to flee Hitler's bunker had carefully avoided on the night of 1 May, was the quickest way out of the centre. Therefore the Russians, well aware of that, concentrated their fire on that area. Just where Api had to turn from Friedrichstrasse east into Ziegelstrasse he saw a large smouldering fire, which the Russians had set at night in order to oversee activities on Friedrichstrasse better. Api also noticed starving people carve up a horse that had died days ago. He himself was hungry most of the time. His daily rations consisted of one slice of bread with margarine and two cups of coffee, or coffee substitute, in the morning, two bowls of thin pea or carrot soup at lunch, and more soup and two slices of bread for dinner.

At 5.30 p.m. that afternoon the first Russians showed up to check out the clinic, its patients, staff and supplies. Typically the Russians had a lot of questions for the staff and the chief physician, and they usually had someone who could speak a little German. '*Du nicht lügen,*' 'You not lie,' they demanded. First they enquired about the clinic, how many beds, what kind of surgical equipment, how much medication. They were particularly interested to find out how many and what kind of weapons the clinic still had, since hand-to-hand fighting continued. They told the doctors to make detailed lists of everything. The Russians also wanted to know who was a member of the Nazi Party and whether any of them ever fought on the Eastern Front. The Germans had committed many atrocities against the Russians there, both military and civilian. Finally they asked about a place to live for their captain and, last but not least, about *Schnapps*, liquor.

As soon as he took over as commander of Berlin, General Nikolai Bersarin tried to control the chaos and establish some sense of normalcy in the city. At age 41, Bersarin was one of the youngest generals in the Soviet army and the best liked by Berliners. Like all medical personnel in Berlin, Api had to register with the Russian authorities. They wanted to compile a list of all doctors in order to set up meetings of health professionals as soon as possible. Api hoped that as a result they would be allowed to move out of the cellars and at least find space for the sick on the first storey of buildings, no matter how damaged. 'Otherwise they are lying around without care and without a roof over their heads. Doctors are still available, only no places to work!'

On the next day, 2 May, the *Wehrmachtsbericht*, the report of the German armed forces, showed itself completely out of touch with reality when it issued this announcement: 'The Führer has died at the head of the courageous defenders of the Reich capital.' That same day at 3 p.m. General Weidling, whom Hitler had appointed commander of Berlin on 23 April, submitted the official capitulation in order to prevent further bloodshed. Weidling stated unequivocally that the Führer had committed suicide and thereby abandoned all who had sworn loyalty to him. He went on to urge everyone to cease resistance at once. Cars with loudspeakers conveyed his message along deserted streets: 'Every hour that you continue to fight only prolongs the terrible suffering of the civilian population and of our wounded. Anyone who still dies fighting for Berlin makes this ultimate sacrifice in vain.' General Weidling, who was not a member of the Nazi Party, ultimately became a Soviet prisoner accused of war crimes and died in a Soviet prison in 1955.

On that same 2 May – although I doubt that Api knew this – ten men arrived in Berlin who were to play a decisive part in its future for decades to come. These were the *Gruppe Ulbricht*, a group of German functionaries of the Communist Party under the leadership of Walter Ulbricht. They returned to Germany from their Russian exile, where they had busied themselves translating propaganda material into German and supporting the Soviet regime in every way they could. Now they were sent back to Germany with the commission to rebuild district administrations in Berlin under Communist guidance. Eventually, Walter Ulbricht became the head of the new German Democratic Republic, the DDR, which he ruled despotically as first secretary of the Socialist Unity Party from 1950 until Chairman Leonid Breshnev forced him to resign in 1971.

On 4 May Api was ordered to report to the post office bunker on Monbijoustrasse at the end of Ziegelstrasse, where help was desperately needed for the many untended injured there. The next morning he packed his rucksack with his few belongings and moved to the cellar of the post office bunker. He found conditions there even worse than what he had experienced so far. He was surrounded by 135 wounded people lying on pallets on the floor. The air stank of their wounds and not much could be done to help the sufferers. And then there were the lice. They crawled everywhere in that dark and mouldy cellar and Api scratched himself all through the night. Later, in the winter of 1945, the health department would issue a poster that warned '*Töte die Laus, sonst tötet sie dich*', 'Kill the louse or it kills you'. Typhus and para typhus were carried by lice.

Api overheard a conversation in the post office bunker that he took down right away. An anxious patient stopped a passing Russian officer to ask: 'What will become of us? Are we going to Siberia?' The Russian responded in his broken but melodious German:

> Nonsense. You go home and you will do the same work you have done so far. The Russian isn't bad and the German isn't bad, but sentimental. *Lumpen* [meaning scoundrels] exist among Russians and Germans alike. And Siberia. With that they only wanted to scare you. What do you think of Siberia? No one eats such black bread there as yours is here.

This officer was typical of many of the Russians who first visited the clinics and bunkers. They were honest and understanding military men who felt sorry for what this terrible war had done, both to their own and to the German people.

The next day, Sunday 6 May, was the first really warm day and Api, who had the day off from the post office bunker, had heard that help was needed to install a military hospital in the former North Sanatorium on Johannisstrasse 10, at the corner of Artelleriestrasse. It was close by, the next street north of Ziegelstrasse. Api knew that the North Sanatorium had been a small private clinic, listed with a capacity of thirty-two beds.

Since as a doctor he had more liberty to move about the streets than the ordinary population, he walked over there to see how he could be of use. It felt good to get out of the dark post office bunker and see the sky. On his way Api took time to observe 'A wonderful morning with a pale blue sky in which swim, almost transparent themselves, the ornaments of the church towers'. The beginning of May was balmy with sunny days and blue skies. The surviving linden trees that lined the streets were a bright green and the dust and rubble on the pavements was covered with their blossoms. Api delighted, as he had always done, in the signs of nature's rebirth. Even though he felt dizzy, feverish and sick to his stomach, just being out of doors and able to look at the sky helped him a little to cope with what lay ahead in labour, pain and mental shock.

The staff at the North Sanatorium welcomed him with open arms. There was so much to be done to ready the place for patients. So every day after he was finished at the post office bunker, Api helped out at the North Sanatorium. There he witnessed a much wilder group of Russian soldiers than had come earlier to the Ziegelstrasse clinic. They were looting the little the doctors had managed to scrape together for their patients. They considered that everything in Berlin was rightfully theirs. 'Private property does not exist. Everything is Soviet property despite their first edict, which made one full of hope, which said that it is forbidden to enter private apartments and to pillage.' Api found a pair of high-laced shoes to replace his army boots, but he did not dare clean them for fear that if they looked too good they would be taken away from him on the street. Over the next weeks the lawlessness and lack of personal security added a heavy burden to his other worries.

Api was becoming increasingly more hopeless and desperate. He felt trapped in Berlin's grey ruins. Moreover the starvation diet, which continued unabated and even got worse, began to take its toll on his energy and his health. But more important than any of this was that as soon as the war had ended Api had one main goal on his mind: to come to us in Suderburg, or at least to let us know that he had survived. Neither was possible. Without permissions or papers, he saw no way of fleeing from Berlin Mitte and undertaking the long journey on foot. And without postal service he could not communicate with us, either. Instead, Api handed letters and postcards to anyone who was trying to get out of Berlin. The first message that made it through did not get to us until 10 September 1945.

At last, on 8 May, came the official declaration in the *Wehrmachtsbericht*, the report of the army high command, that beginning at midnight on 9 May all fighting was to cease. By that time no resistance was left. This announcement followed the signing of the military surrender with the Allies and the Red Army at midnight on 8 May. It took place in the new Soviet headquarters in Karlshorst on the south-eastern edge of Berlin. The Second World War was finally and officially over. The army high command ended its records with this bow to the millions of dead: 'In this difficult hour the armed forces commemorate their comrades lost before the enemy. The dead demand unconditional loyalty, obedience, and discipline for the fatherland which is bleeding from innumerable wounds.'

The 9 May was declared the Day of Victory by the Soviets and outbreaks of shooting from machine guns, flak stations, tanks and pistols scared Berliners anew, but they were only 'salutes to peace'. Today, more than sixty years later, Germans often call 9 May the Day of Liberation, although it was not seen that way by those who lived through it at the time.

23

My Painful Hour

Take good care of our littlest sunshine and
occasionally tell her of her poor Api's heartrending
longing ... But yet leave her some sunshine which she
needs for the development of her little soul.

Now that the war was finally over, Api gathered what little
emotional and physical energy he had to think about
rebuilding his practice and creating a footing for our future.
His role as the sole supporter of our family had always been
his pride and ambition, but now it both helped him to hold out and added
additional stress. Trying to find a way to support his family forced him not
to give up and even at times buoyed him, with thoughts of a once again
happy future together. He dreamt that he could start again as he had done
in 1920. At the same time, it also drove him to despair, for he did not know
how to accomplish this one supremely important goal of his life and feared
that he no longer was up to the job. He wondered what start was possible
among nothing but ruins and beggars when 'we have lost everything
without exception'.

The mornings and evenings were Api's hardest times. Yet he always
got up at 6 a.m. 'only so that I can give myself for one hour to my painful
longing'. He reviewed the many happy times of his life: his poor but happy

childhood in Marienwerder, the early days of his marriage, the birth of his children, right up to his weekend visits to us in Joachimsthal during 1944 to where we had fled for a time when we were bombed out. Api had to remain behind in the city and could visit only rarely. He thought about the many coffee hours on the balcony, the music they made and the life they built. Thinking all that was forever lost steeped him in despair and longing. During the rest of the day Api had little time to worry about his situation, since every minute was taken up with hard labour. From 8 a.m., the time the curfew ended, to 8 p.m. without rest he assisted in small operations, did surgical dressings and saw patients. Without medications, food and still insufficient places to bed them, he could not do enough for them and felt helpless in the face of their suffering. He was particularly affected by starving babies and their sick mothers for whom he was unable to provide nourishment.

In addition to medical work, Api also laboured physically. The military hospital in the North Sanatorium still needed so much. He hauled furniture and foraged for medications and dressing materials in all kinds of devastated places. He explored abandoned medical cellars and gingerly climbed broken stairs to former supply rooms. Wherever he went he had to be careful not to step on broken glass or sharp bits of metal, all of which lay buried under thick layers of dust, which made it hard to breathe. His clothes and hair became impregnated with it and the pores of his skin were caked with it, plastered down by sweat. The weather had turned oppressively hot and the plague of lice made his dry and dirty skin itch unbearably.

To his delight, on 10 May Api was given permission to leave the post office bunker and settle in the North Sanatorium. For the first time in weeks he had a place to stay above ground; in fact he was given an attic room four stories up. Of the two small windows in his room, one was half cardboard, the other open altogether – but at least he could breathe fresh air and see the sky. As soon as he stepped inside his new home he rushed to the window and drew in deep breaths, although the air was still tinged with smoke and dust. Except for the clouds and the birds, the view that met him was most depressing. He looked out on the burnt rafters of a bombed-out roof directly across from him. All the other buildings had no roofs at all, they were just a sea of grey ruins and only here and there did a church spire still reach out of the rubble.

On the first full day in his attic room, Api celebrated the occasion by giving himself a thorough wash even though he had only cold water which he had to carry in. It was difficult to rub the dust and grime out of his pores and his hair, but the wash did him good. He felt cleaner than he had in weeks. Afterwards he put on fresh underwear, which in itself was a luxury. He brushed and shook out his army shirt and pants which he had worn for weeks. But since he had no other clothing he had to make do with them again. As a final layer, he pulled out of his rucksack a blue-grey sweater, which once had belonged to Nyussi. It had accompanied him during the worst days of his son's death as well as the happy moments in Suderburg. It had become to him a symbol of her love and loyalty and he never put it on without kissing it first.

Feeling clean and protected, Api sat down near the open window and took out his diary. From then on he would spend every free minute by his attic window dreaming of freedom and a reunion. In his most desperate moments it helped him to gaze out on the city and scan the sky, noting the shapes of the clouds and the flight of the swallows, and delight in how the sun painted the torn and bent rafters a golden red. He then recorded it all in his diary. Studying sky and clouds became his respite of meditation even if it often ended in desperate longing. With his belief in always being purposeful, he thought 'that all this conjuring up of sweetest thoughts is useless and lost time, but for me it is uplifting'.

Wrapped in Nyussi's sweater, Api began that evening by reporting on the sky. He concentrated on being as descriptive as he could be. Yet words no longer came as easily as before, and he felt that even language, which always had been so important in his life, was now deserting him. As he started to write, he imagined that he was talking to us and making us see what he saw, then the words flowed more easily:

On a pale blue evening sky big bellied and deformed wind clouds are spread in a colourless light. Through it race, screeching, a few swifts (many don't have any possibility of nesting since everything is rubble and ashes.) Smoke columns from new fires still rise somewhere above the ruins of the roofs, sometimes thinner, sometimes thicker. The warm air is heavy with dust and smoke.

A barking dog in the area made Api stop for a moment and think of the Hungarian sheep dog Ficko, which just means 'dog', in Nyussi's home town Nagykörös and the 'blessed times' they all had enjoyed there. Then he listened to someone across the street who was playing on an out-of-tune piano, which made him even sadder:

> We will certainly not make music any more ... And yet if only the family and the enjoyment of God's wonderful nature remain for us. How I would pray and work in humble thankfulness! ... But perhaps I love you even more now than then, that is, more consciously aware that you are my one and all in this world ... If only one were free!! Freedom, health, a bicycle for which I would give gold – and off to you!!!

A map of Germany was always on his bedside table and his eyes often measured the distance of about 150 miles from Berlin to Uelzen, the district capital. Suderburg was too small to be listed, but he marked the spot where it should have been with a little cross. Seeing the very name of Uelzen on that map made him break down in yearning and despair.

In a spare moment on Monday 14 May, when the air had cleared after a heavy night storm, Api went back to the Luisenstrasse cellar to fetch the only clothes left to him, so that he could delouse what he had been living in for all this time. After the fourth-floor apartment had been destroyed, Api had stored some of his belongings in the cellar. That is also where he put his son's bike. He had made sure to take out the valves to prevent theft. Now he carefully climbed down the stairs to the cellar, stepping over heaps of plaster with crunching broken glass beneath his shoes. With each step his feet sank into the fine, chalk-like dust that covered everything in the city. When he reached the door of his section of the cellar, he found the lock broken. Looking inside he saw that everything was gone. He particularly missed the suitcase in which he had stored all his papers, poems and diaries. I, too, am sorry that I have only a handful of letters and poems of what must have been hundreds of pieces of writing – for Api recorded everything. Most of what I have dates from after 1945. They are poems and thoughts for our birthdays, for Advent, Christmas, the New Year, for the seasons on the heath, the blossoming of spring and the fogs of autumn. So I can imagine that, in addition to diaries, he had a similar collection for all the years up to 1945. Looking at the empty cellar, however, Api was most devastated by the loss of his son's bicycle, on which he had set such hope. It was to be his way out of Berlin and to us.

Yet Api also knew that he could not leave and that even if with extraordinary luck he should get out of Berlin without being stopped, shot or having his bike stolen, he would not be able to cross the River Elbe, the wide river that formed part of the dividing line between the Soviet occupation zone and those of the Western Allies. Api had heard rumours of hundreds of refugees dying in the attempt to get across the Elbe. It was said people either drowned in the river or were killed by the Allies on the bridge. But despite all this, the loss of the bike was a physical reminder of his imprisonment and how impossible it was for him to move.

I remember as a child standing at the shores of the broad Elbe near Hamburg, not far from where it flows into the North Sea. I was on the western side and looked across to the ominous wooden watchtowers that had been erected all along the eastern shore. Occasionally I caught a glimpse of an armed patrol. To me the *Ostzone*, the Eastern Zone, was a forbidden land of mystery and danger. Still today, more than fifteen years after reunification, I cannot get used to the ease with which Mike and I drive into the former East Germany. There is just a sign on the Autobahn telling us that this is where East Germany began, and we notice that the highway is newer from then on. What had been to me a forbidden country when I was growing up is now just a smooth uninterrupted stretch of Autobahn.

Feeling even more hopeless about reaching us now that the bike was gone, on his way back from the apartment Api noticed signs which showed that he was not alone in his desperate worry about relatives. Hastily written messages on bits of paper were stuck to door frames or pinned to a lamppost. Some said that they had survived and could be found at this new address. Others asked for information about the occupants of one of the flats in what was now a gaping hole or a heap of stones. Mothers were looking for their sons who had served in the *Volkssturm*, the People's Militia, and had not been heard from since. People had no other way of communicating than through these scraps of paper; so many messages, each with its own desperate story and little hope of a happy ending.

125

When Api climbed the stairs up to his attic, a patient from the North Sanatorium was waiting at his door. Knowing how much Api would enjoy it, he offered him a bouquet of lilies of the valley and a few stalks of lilac he had picked out of the ruins. Any sign of nature softened Api's despair and kindled his love, and also his love of words. He was grateful that the patient had taken the trouble of bringing these gifts of spring to him:

> The lilies of the valley are fragrant on my little table. The lilac stands in my attic window with the pale blue evening sky in the background above which radiant pink wind clouds drift northeast in a barely perceptible movement, a symbol of the most distant, the most delicate, unfulfillable dreams of peace and happiness under a heaven of divine infinity and steady goodness.

Despite this momentary peaceful vision, the anxiety about us and about the future began to weigh on Api more and more. He slept badly and suffered from night sweats, and during the day he had dizzy spells and felt feverish. Sleep was difficult because of constant noise in the streets where Russian soldiers were shooting almost as if the war was still raging. Yet Api could not afford to be tired. In addition to medical work, he had errands to run. First of all, he needed a certificate to show that he was working for the public health department. He also wanted to make sure that it said, as was the case, that he was doing this without obligation, so that he could start a private practice. Perhaps Api thought back to his controversy with the Charité over setting up his own practice and wanted to avoid a similar conflict. In order to get this certificate he first had to go to chief army physician Dr Kleberger, who was in charge of the North Sanatorium, and then to the mayor. I am not sure but assume that this was the chief mayor of Berlin, Dr Arthur Werner, whom Bersarin had just appointed. His office was in the *Neues Stadthaus*, the New City Hall, which had not been badly damaged. It was located on Parochialstrasse south of Unter den Linden in Berlin Mitte, a hike of about an hour. Api was glad that he did not have to go quite as far as Alexanderplatz, which was growing into a centre for black marketeers. Cigarettes were the currency that got one access to anything: old shoes, herrings, used clothes and even a little Nescafé.

On his way, Api for the first time noticed long columns of women, their heads wrapped in kerchiefs, working in the streets. They were known as the *Trümmerfrauen*, the rubble women. For eight hours every day they passed buckets of stones from hand to hand in a human chain. They salvaged what bricks were still usable by cleaning off the old cement and stacking them in neat rows. Hundreds of thousands of bricks were restored in this way from what seemed like an inexhaustible supply. Berlin Mitte alone had 127 million cubic feet of rubble. Altogether 6 square miles of the city had been levelled, creating 3 billion cubic feet of rubble. Except for the *Trümmerfrauen*, Api saw few people roaming around the mountains of crumbled and dusty stones.

Once he got the certificate he needed, Api turned his mind seriously to rebuilding his practice. His young colleague Dr Heinz Kraaz offered to come along to Luisenstrasse to see what could be done there. For hours Dr Kraaz swept and shovelled with a true joy in helping – although they almost suffocated from the layers of dust they stirred up. Api was grateful for the young man's help, and even more so for his encouraging presence. He knew now that he could not have stayed there by himself. Alone, without this friendly support, he would have given up in despair, especially when he came across bits and pieces of his past. At one point he found pictures of me, which that evening inspired him to write: 'Take good care of our littlest sunshine and occasionally tell her of her poor Api's heartrending longing ... But yet leave her some sunshine which she needs for the development of her little soul.'

It was from the middle of May onwards, about two weeks after the end of the war and the beginning of the Russian occupation, that Api's courage seriously began to desert him. So far he had struggled on, first in the hope that the war would end soon, then that the Americans would come and alleviate the Russian occupation. When that failed, he still hoped that he would be able to travel to Suderburg soon and, taking us all with him, start his practice again in his old home in Berlin. But none of this happened as he had imagined it. He was trapped in a devastated city without any hope of seeing us ever again.

Api felt so hopeless that for the first time in his life the thought of suicide began to haunt him, although he never called it that directly in his diary. On Thursday night, 17/18 May, he made the first oblique reference:

I do not know what will happen. Never before have I felt so close to this step, so compellingly close! Hopelessness, loneliness, bleakness, boundless desolation, and direct danger with 100,000 screaming and terrible voices which drown out the memory of the sweetest harmony and blissful contentment. Gone! Gone for all times.

A heavy thunderstorm, accompanied by such a wind that he feared his little attic would fly away, seemed to echo his desperate and tumultuous thoughts. He finally took *Bromural*, a heavy sleeping powder, to help him through the night.

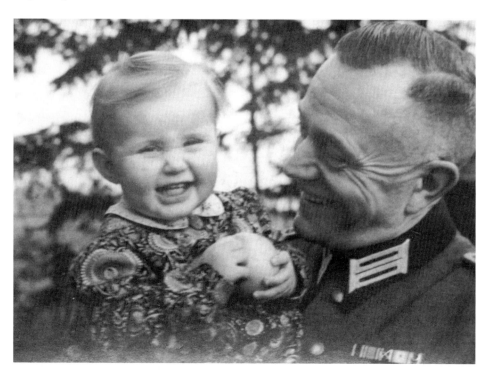

1 Api's diary.

2 Api and I.

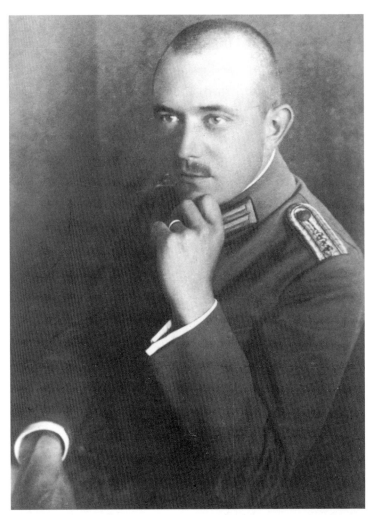

3 Api in the First World War.

4 Döhrmann family; my grandmother second from left.

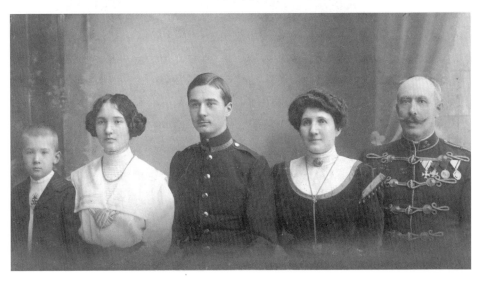

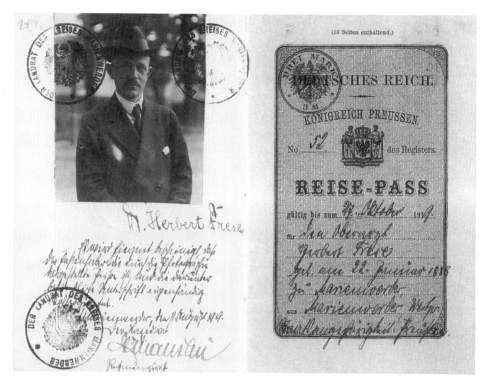

5 Passport from a vanished kingdom.

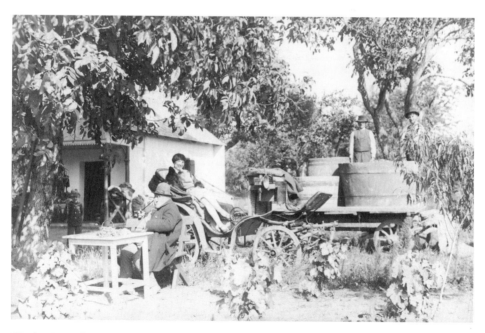

6 In the vineyards in Hungary.

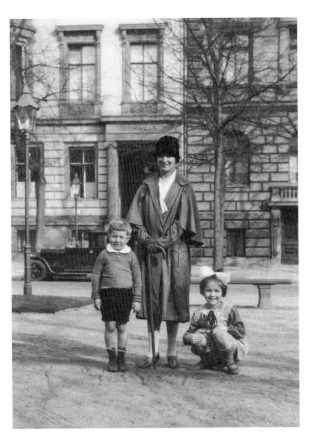

7 Nyussi and her children in front of their Luisenstrasse apartment.

8 Luisenstrasse in 2008.

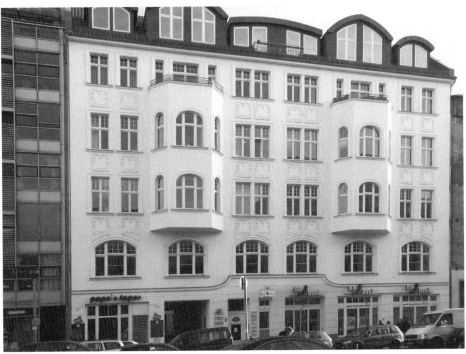

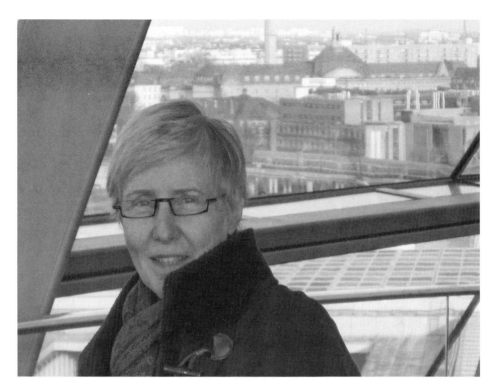

9 On top of the Reichstag with the Emperor Wilhelm Academy in the background, where Api was a medical student.

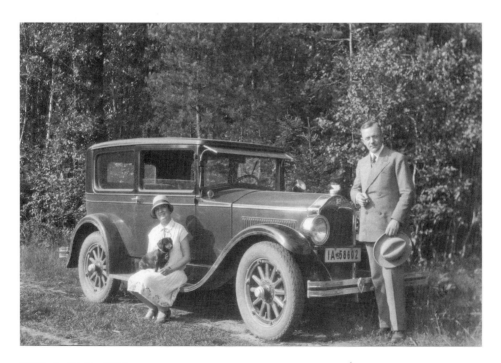

10 The first Buick, 1926.

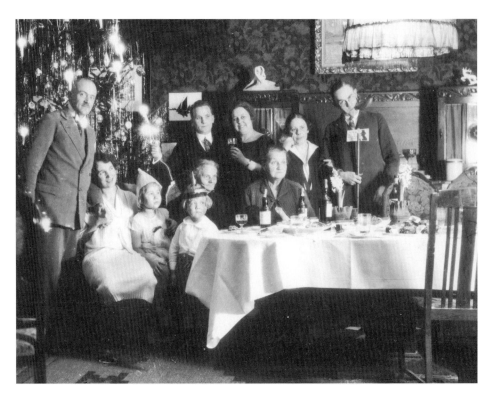

11 Christmas 1927: Api, Nyussi, my mother and uncle on left.

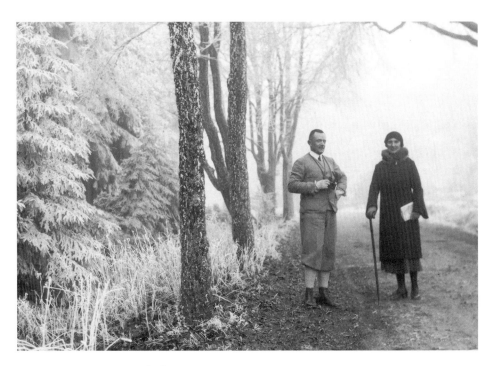

12 Api and Nyussi in the Riesengebirge.

13 A memorial postcard from 1933, when Hitler became chancellor.

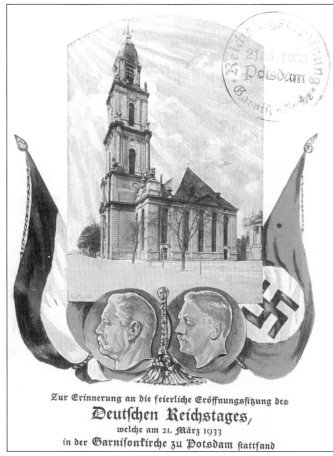

Zur Erinnerung an die feierliche Eröffnungssitzung des

Deutschen Reichstages,

welche am 21. März 1933
in der Garnisonkirche zu Potsdam stattfand

14 Nyussi and her children in Unter den Linden, 1936.

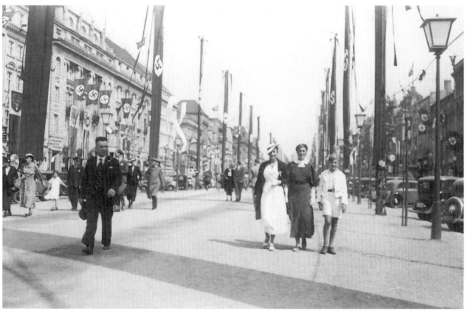

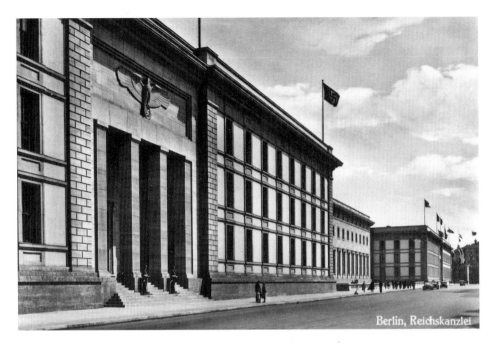

15 Postcard of the New Reichs Chancellery.

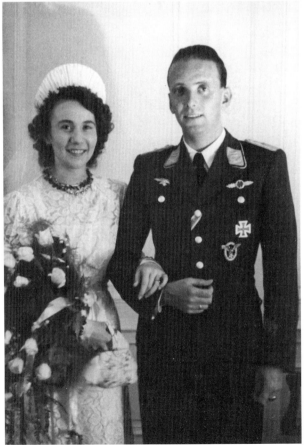

16 My parents' wedding, 29 September 1941.

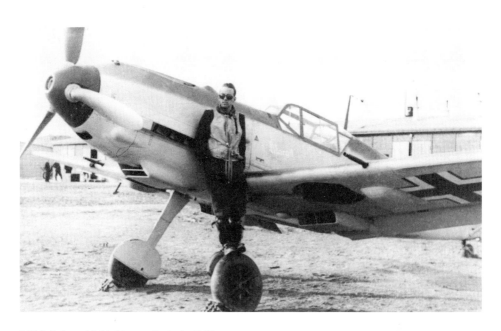

17 My father with his Messerschmitt in 1942.

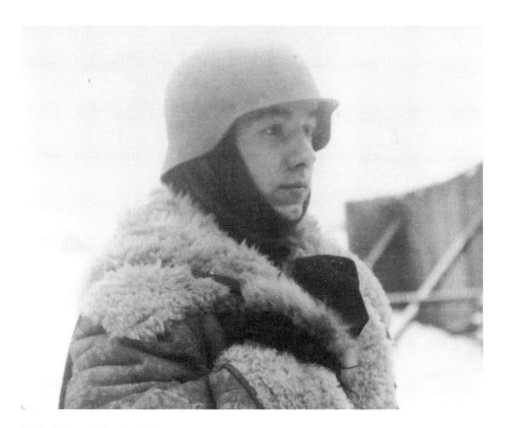

18 Uncle Dieter in Russia, 1942.

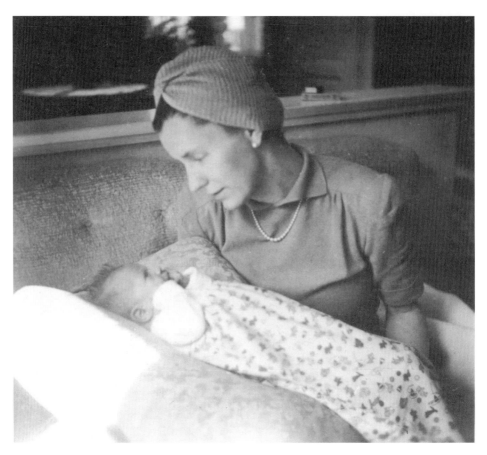

19 My mother and I, October 1942.

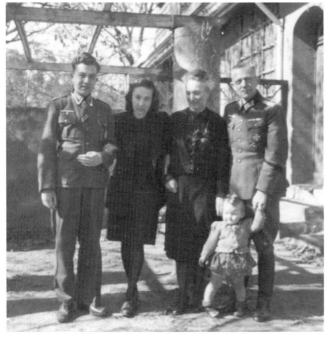

20 Uncle Dieter, my mother, Nyussi, Api and I in Joachimsthal after my father's death, 1943.

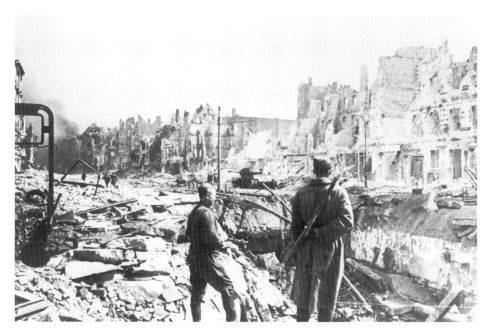

21 Berlin, May 1945. (Courtesy bpk-Bildagentur für Kunst, Kultur und Geschichte, #30015607)

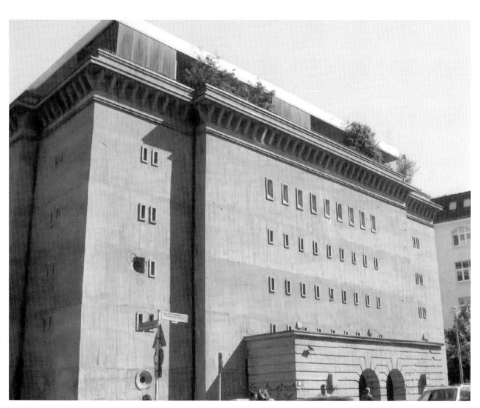

22 The Albrechtstrasse Bunker in 2008, now a museum of contemporary art.

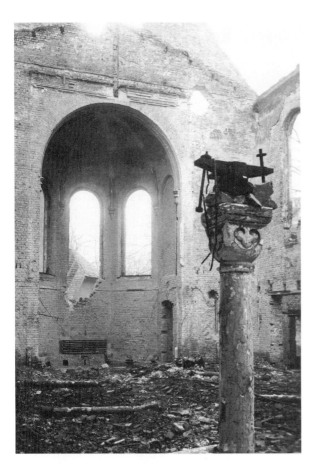

23 Philippus Apostel church, 1945. (Courtesy Landeskirchliches Archiv Berlin ELAB Bestand 7.1 2346 from the collection Stephani)

24 The Suderburg church.

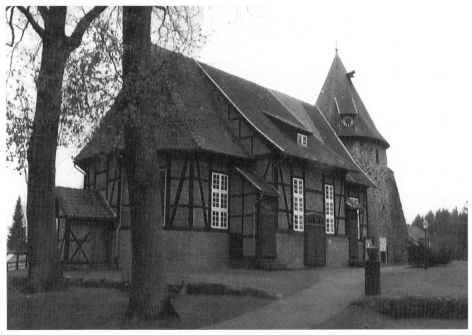

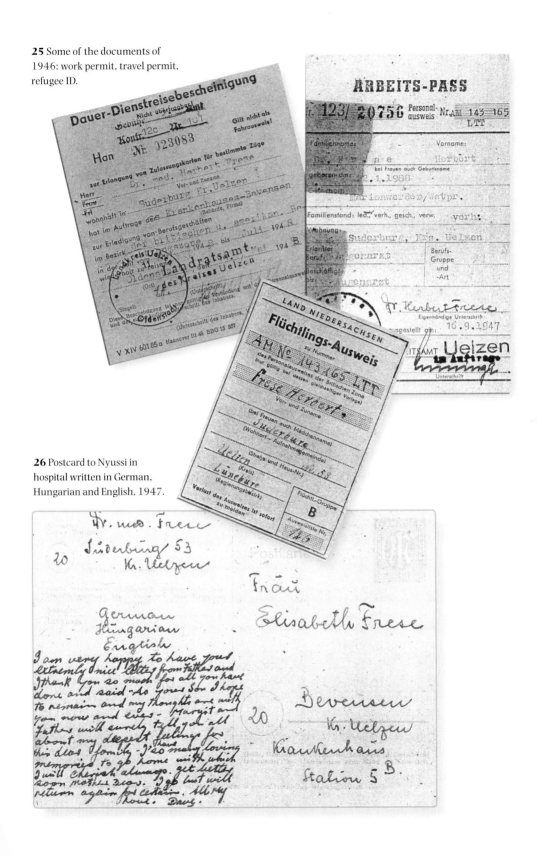

25 Some of the documents of 1946: work permit, travel permit, refugee ID.

26 Postcard to Nyussi in hospital written in German, Hungarian and English, 1947.

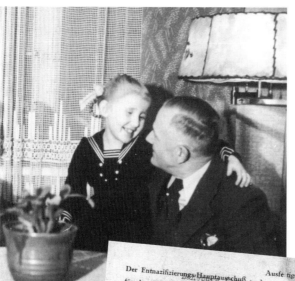

27 Api and I in the Bevensen apartment, 1949.

28 Api's de-Nazification document, 1949.

Der Entnazifizierungs-Hauptausschuß　Ausfetigung
für den Kreis

(24a) Lüneburg (Landgericht)

Az. H.VE
SpF 418

Lüneburg, den
Am Mark 7 (Landgericht)
Fernsprecher: 5282, 4873, 4974, 4878

19. Mai 1949

19. Mai 1949

gez. Höffer

Rechtskräftig am:

Lüneburg, den

ger.

[Geschäftsstellenleiter]

Entnazifizierungs-Entscheidung im schriftlichen Verfahren.

In dem Entnazifizierungsverfahren gegen

Name **F r e s e**   Herbert

geboren am 22.1.1888   Vornamen Marienwerder/Westpr.

wohnhaft Suderburg 55 Kreis Uelzen

Beruf **Arzt/Augenarzt**

ergeht auf Antrag des Öffentlichen Klägers bei den Entnazifizierungs-Hauptausschüssen
im Regierungs-Bezirk Lüneburg Az. Lbg. (Aerzte)   19.5.1949 vom

auf Grund der Verordnung über Rechtsgrundsätze der Entnazifizierung im Lande
Niedersachsen vom 3. 7. 1948 und § 19 der Verordnung über das Verfahren zur
Fortführung und zum Abschluß der Entnazifizierung im Lande Niedersachsen vom
30. 3. 1948 im schriftlichen Verfahren folgende Entscheidung:

1. **Der Betroffene wird gemäss § 7 (1)a als
   entlastet (Kategorie V)
   eingestuft.**

2. Die Kosten des Verfahrens, einschl. Auslagen, werden auf DM 20,-- festgesetzt

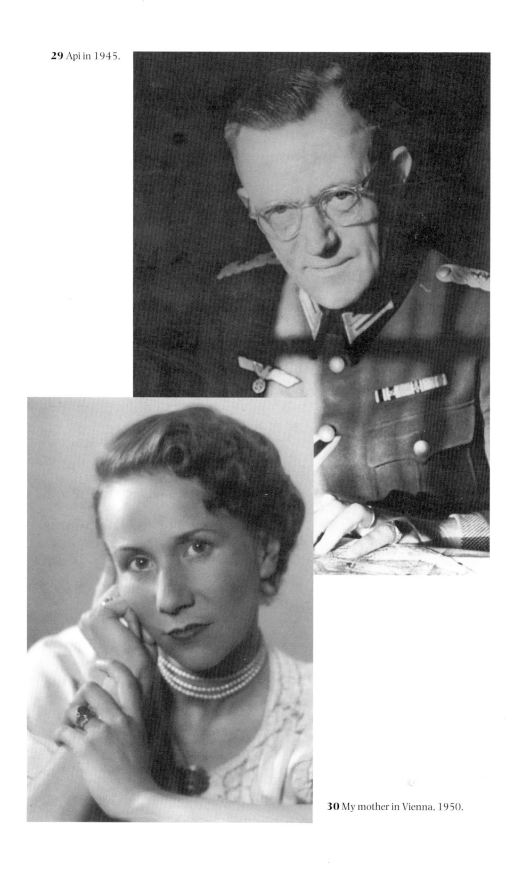

29 Api in 1945.

30 My mother in Vienna, 1950.

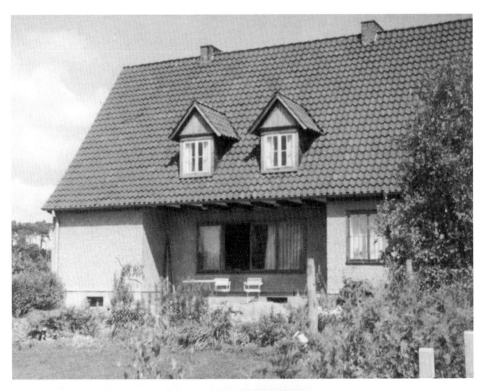

31 The house in Bevensen.

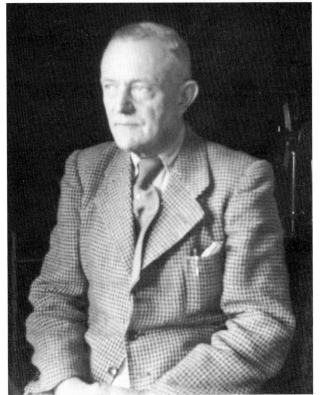

32 Api in 1950, wearing his favorite pearl tiepin.

24

Pentecost Sunday

Oh, how close I was to you and with what desperate longing did I think of our last church visit in Suderburg. Blessed, blessed time!

On Saturday 19 May, Api obtained a certificate of military discharge from Professor Ferdinand Sauerbruch of the Charité, who from May to October 1945 served on the Berlin City Council for Health. Thus relieved of his military responsibilities, Api felt freer and decided to take a walk in search of a church for next day's Pentecost Sunday. The streets were deserted and he hardly met a soul the entire time. He looked into the ruins of churches and saw organ pipes lying about, and burial chambers and subterranean vaults broken into. He so loved to hear an organ play in church, but none of the ones he saw that afternoon would play again. Although the sky was cloudless, it was veiled in smoke and the stench of corpses brooded unbearably beneath it.

On Pentecost Sunday, the descent of the Holy Spirit, Api could not bear to be alone with his thoughts. It had always been such a bright, joyful holiday at the beginning of spring. So he went to look for his two friends, Sister Briese and Sister Baesler, both deaconesses whom he had met at the North Sanatorium. They were not the Nazi deaconesses who had sworn their oath of loyalty to Hitler instead of Jesus, but the traditional Protestant ones. Much like Catholic nuns, these Protestant sisters lived together in mother houses where they shared a simple life. Each order had its own habit, although they all wore stiff white caps ruffled at the back, mostly grey or blue shirts with white collars, and a short tunic. Their only decoration was a broach or a chain with a cross and the insignia of their order. Api had always felt close to the deaconesses he had known whose mission it was to serve others, particularly the sick. He shared their strong Lutheranism and respected their dedication. At the North Sanatorium Api had come to love the two sisters who visited every day from their mother house on nearby Tieckstrasse to help out wherever they could.

When I lived with my grandparents after the war, they continued to befriend the local deaconesses. Many a time I came in from play to see one of these elderly ladies in her white cap having coffee with Api and Nyussi, who always served special treats and cakes for them. As I greeted her with a curtsey, I always was struck by the little cape she had around her shoulders. To me it looked as if she had stepped out of a fairy tale. But then my formal curtsey now seems to me to be part of another world as well, although I remember that I greeted adults with curtseys well into my teenage years.

Together Api and the two deaconesses set out to find a church that still had a playable organ. They walked to the end of Ziegelstrasse immediately east of Monbijou Park, where just a few days ago Api had watched the chief physician stack corpses. They passed the old Jewish cemetery that had been destroyed by the Nazis in 1943. Now the cemetery was used to bury the many dead of the neighbourhood. The adjacent red-brick synagogue had been damaged in Kristallnacht back in 1938. Two blocks east of there, only a fifteen-minute walk altogether, stood the Sophien church, the head church of the parish where Api had been an elder. Api was delighted when he saw that the Sophien church still had its organ intact. The three of them sat in a pew with a small group of other ragged and care-worn people, looking out of the broken windows on to blackened trees. As the organ began, Api's thoughts drifted westward to Suderburg and a much smaller, tree-shaded church:

Oh, how close I was to you and with what desperate longing did I think of our last church visit in Suderburg. Blessed, blessed time!

The devotion was a high edification and at the same time such a
mental stress that one could hardly master one's tears.

Api's imagination pictured us walking through the village toward the
brick-and-timber church with its medieval tower of rough grey stone.
The church stood so clearly before his eyes, the old red brick set off by age-
darkened timbers, the three long, white-paned windows on each side and
the incongruous grey tower where Herr Klapproth, the Ohlde's neighbour,
rang the bells. He thought that we had just about reached the ancient
village square to greet the old church where it stood surrounded by tall
and gnarled oak trees. The weather was ideal for a journey west. Five days
on foot should bring him to the River Elbe, and then two more after that if,
despite all reports to the contrary, he was lucky enough to get across. Yet he
dared not risk it.

Of course, Mike and I also paid a visit to Sophien church. It has the most
beautiful baroque onion spire in all of Berlin, which had beckoned to us and
shown us the way with its delicate green-and-gold copper tower. We found
the church sequestered in its own small churchyard shaded by linden trees.
The trees were old, and I wondered whether any of them had been there
in 1945. An 8ft-high ornate iron railing separates the church grounds
from the quiet neighbourhood of tree-lined streets and apartment houses.
When we walked on we found other places Api had mentioned in the diary.
The large, red-brick Hedwig's Hospital is still there around the corner from
the church and we saw how close the synagogue, also built of red brick,
was. The whole area exuded a subdued calm and repose, but it also felt left
behind the times. Part of the former East Berlin, it had not yet caught up
with the busy commercialism of the West. In contrast to the streets west of
Kurfürstendamm, we saw no restaurants, wine bars and bakeries, and very
few people.

After church Api decided to make use of this holiday to do more cleaning
in his surgery. He managed to rid the small green consulting room of most
of the dirt, wash the dented and bent instruments and scrub the chairs
and the desk so he could use them. The windows, of course, were all
broken and glass unavailable. There also was no electricity, without which
his surgery could not function. Nevertheless, he did not give up hope that
he would be able to hold office hours again soon. He made up his mind

to look for new instruments. His bank accounts and savings certificates were gone, but he had some cash left. At some time in the middle of May, I do not know exactly when, Api put most of that money into the reconstruction of his practice. In his diary he justified this action, which also kept him in Berlin: 'I had to make the effort. That also is the reason – among others – why I decided to stay. God grant that it was right.'

Although Api did not mention it, and perhaps he did not know, on that Pentecost Sunday, 20 May, while he was busy in his surgery, a new Berlin City Council had been formed in the New City Hall he had visited a few days earlier. The council was dominated by the Communists, who held 100 out of 230 seats. Even if he heard this news, he could not have foreseen that this was the beginning of the totalitarian rule which presided over East Berlin and the entire Communist German Democratic Republic, the DDR, until the fall of the Berlin Wall in 1989.

When he returned to his attic he found a piece of cake on his table: a gift from the nurses at the North Sanatorium who helped him whenever they could. Throughout his career Api had been on excellent terms with nurses. He was cordial, considerate and charming. They knew how much he valued them and they liked that he could make them laugh even amidst the worst pressures. So they tried to look after him as well. It was their caring as much as the food that sustained Api in his loneliness. After he had eaten the cake, he fetched twelve pails of water for the special treat of a bath.

Api ended his Pentecost Sunday by the attic window. He gazed out at a clear silver half-moon and wondered whether, at this very moment, we were enjoying the same sight out of our cottage window. As he contemplated that sliver of moon, a smile spread across his weary face. He was thinking about an argument he had had with my mother about the moons. She was small, not yet in school. Looking out their living room window she saw a bright and fully rounded moon lighting up the courtyard. She ran quickly to the kitchen at the front of the apartment and yes, there was another, just as round and bright, shedding its silver light on the street below. With such incontrovertible evidence she refused to believe her father's explanation that there was only one moon in the sky.

25

A Little Light

If peace and rest would come at last!! An indescribably
beautiful and peaceful evening sky and the poor earth
torn apart in hostility and destruction, in enmity and
hatred, in impossibility for life and in misery.

O n Pentecost Monday Api arranged with a Herr Küssner to have
a special memorial for his dead son Dieter. Api often mentioned
the name Küssner in his diary in connection with the Charité
chapel, but I had no luck finding him in their extensive archives.
Finally Dr Karin Köhler, archivist at the Landeskirchliche Archiv on
Bethaniendamm in Berlin Kreuzberg, helped me out. We went there on
the morning of the UEFA Euro 2008 final in June. We had avoided going
from west to east on the subways, but even the taxi had trouble getting
around the milling tens of thousands of fans. Once we reached the area of
Bethaniendamm, however, the streets were empty.

We found the archives in a new building just off the avenue. The reading
room looked out on a park and a children's playground. Dr Köhler met me
with a stack of papers, saying she hoped I would find what I needed here. It
did not take me long to see Küssner's name. Not surprisingly, he had been
the minister at the Philippus Apostel church, where Api had been an elder.
The pastor had known my grandparents since 1924 when they moved to

Luisenstrasse and he was an assistant minister. Ernst Küssner was born in Berlin in 1878, ten years before Api, and like him had studied at Friedrich Wilhelm University. He was ordained in 1905 and appointed at Philippus Apostel church in 1916, first as assistant, then as second pastor and in 1935 as first pastor. In the records I even found Api's name as member of the church council. The council met at Albrechtstrasse 15, not far from the bunker and my mother's elementary school.

The church archives had pictures of the Philippus Apostle church, both as it had been before the war and how it looked after the bombing, before it was demolished altogether. Today there is no trace left of that church. It had been a largely unremarkable neo-Gothic building of grey stone built at the end of the nineteenth century. The one thing that struck me as unusual was its square spire. After the bombing only the bottom of the tower and one crumbling wall were left standing. This explained why Pastor Küssner held services in the Charité chapel and yet I was unable to locate him through their archives. In the immediate post-war days, pastors could preach in almost any church that was still intact enough to allow it. So Pastor Küssner, whose own church lay in ruins, helped out in the nearby Charité chapel on Luisenstrasse at the western edge of the Charité campus. The chapel had not escaped the bombs but it could still be used.

The memorial for my uncle was not all Api discussed with his pastor friend. He also broached the question of whether a Christian was ever allowed to take his own life. Api did not record the pastor's answer, but I can imagine that it was an absolute 'no'. Api ended by telling Pastor Küssner that if things went badly he would make sure Küssner got his diary to preserve for us.

On Tuesday 22 May Api was a little buoyed by small bits of progress and not even the heavy rain that day could dampen his mood. The first piece of good news was that for one day the mayor's office, anxious to have more medical care, provided him with six women to help clean out the surgery and make two rooms ready to receive patients. On top of that he also managed to get some electrical supplies and even the promise of an electrician to install them. The man told him that he could bring in electricity from the building next door. With electric light, Api could really start to see patients. The electrician showed up the very next day as promised. Once he had made the repairs and light came up in the rooms,

Api, too, felt a surge of energy. Even better, he discovered that much of his expensive equipment still worked. The electrician wanted to be of further help and started to dismantle a broken light above the mirror in the entrance hall. Api rushed to stop him. The light had been installed by my Uncle Dieter. Clinging to the last tokens of his son's presence, he became almost ferocious:

> I had to intervene almost with force. Every time I switch it on, I think
> of his love which made him put this together for me, I see and feel his
> beloved little strong paws. Oh my good boy. If I could get your advice
> now, I would probably follow it since I have such great trust in your
> decisions as I have lost now in my own.

Api was fortunate also in his hunt for other treasures, which were so very hard to obtain in those days. He found a bit of cardboard, a piece of glass and even some nails. In this he was particularly lucky for nails were almost impossible to get anywhere, even on the black market. The apartment, however, still had no running water. He had to carry water in from the police barracks nearby whose garden was dug up for mass graves. As he walked his district, he now could hear a radio playing here and there, although he himself still had only rumours for news. Some of the rumours made him afraid, especially when they hinted at a possible serious conflict between the Russians and the Western Allies, which would mean no resolution to the situation in Berlin.

On Wednesday Api had a row with chief physician of the North Sanatorium, Dr Kleberger, which shook him badly. In what my grandfather thought had been an amicable conversation the day before, Dr Kleberger and he had agreed that there was no longer enough volunteer work for him to do at the North Sanatorium and that he needed to find a living for himself. Now the chief physician denied having said anything of the sort. Api felt as if his life was going in crazy circles and he had returned to the problem with the Charité at the very beginning of his career, but now he was much less able to handle it.

Both Api and Dr Kleberger were certain that they were right. So they looked for confirmation from the person in charge of health in Berlin Mitte, and that was Professor Sauerbruch. When they got to the Charité they were told that the professor was in an operation. Dr Kleberger waited right there but Api, unwisely it seems, left for an appointment. When he returned two hours later, Dr Kleberger had already talked to Professor Sauerbruch and Api did not doubt that he had given a one-sided report. Trying to write away his agitation, Api recollected that Dr Kleberger was not popular with the other doctors. 'He always kept his plans a secret from us. Even things which would have been important. Dr K once told him directly that, after all, one has to do something to get on for oneself since he is making no arrangements whatsoever.' Api then remembered an episode which had made all the doctors angry with the chief physician. One morning Dr Kleberger had told them that it was out of the question for them to appear in civilian clothes. Two days later, however, Dr Kleberger himself did just that to the amazement of his staff:

> He told us that after all everyone is wearing civilian clothes now except for those who are not able to do so! [Probably meaning because they did not have any] ... at any rate, he always was uncomradely, egoism personified. – But let's leave that.

In his fragile state, Api found it hard to forget this altercation, although nothing came of the matter. He was allowed to stay in the attic and help out at the clinic, but the uncertainty of the unresolved situation worried him for the rest of his stay in Berlin.

The days and nights at the end of May passed in what had become a routine of ups and downs; small successes and a little hope for the immediate present followed by despondency about the future. Api still occupied the attic of the sanatorium since he could not yet live in his surgery. One room was almost ready to be turned into his waiting room – even though it had a large hole in the wall and no door. Outside, the city still throbbed with heavy explosions as the Red Army blew up unstable buildings and bridges, and thick clouds of dust and smoke hovered over the centre. No public transport was working in the inner city so that he had to do every errand on foot and, more importantly, could not imagine how patients would be able to reach him. And, of course, Api continued to question himself whether he should try to make the trip to Suderburg. He calculated the various ways: 'half an hour's flight, 6 hours by car, 5 hours by train, 2 days by bike, 7 days on foot. None of it a problem if one only were allowed to go.' If the nights were too bad, Api took *Allional*, a sleeping pill, to slip into oblivion.

Like the smoke hovering over the city, the cloud of loneliness and anxiety about us never left him. He always tried to picture what we might be doing, but he did not even know what time we were on. Berlin had been switched to Moscow time, which was one hour later than the summer time we might be on in Suderburg, and two hours later if we were on Middle European time. This possible two-hour difference, small as it was, troubled him when he tried to imagine our daily activities.

The end of May was as cold as its beginning had been hot. Temperatures stayed below 10°C (50°F). New rumours raised Api's level of anxiety. One in particular upset him and made him recall the disagreement with Dr Kleberger. He heard that military discharges that had been issued by Professor Sauerbruch, as his had been, were not legally binding. Api had no idea whether there was any truth in this and, if so, what it meant for his position. Would he be classified as a deserter? If he was, what should or could he do about it? In the end he felt too enervated and exhausted to do anything or even dwell on the implications of what might, after all, only have been empty gossip. Instead, Api returned over and over to the perennial question in his mind. How could he get to Suderburg? His rucksack was always packed, ready to go, but he did not leave. He had imagined that if only the war was over, everything would get better. Now, however, the occupation brought a whole new set of terrors which, added to the strain of six years of war and twelve years of tyranny, sapped his strength and resolve. It reduced him to a bundle of fear.

The futility of Api's present existence was brought home to him again on Saturday 26 May, when the Russians tried to blow up the bridge in front of the Emperor Friedrich Museum, today called the Bode Museum, on the Museum Island a few blocks east of where Api was. The heavy detonations blew out the one window he just had managed to install.

That evening at his attic window, he wrote by the failing light:

If peace and rest would come at last!! An indescribably beautiful and peaceful evening sky and the poor earth torn apart in hostility and destruction, in enmity and hatred, in impossibility for life and in misery. I do not know how it looks elsewhere and recognize also that it is a near superhuman task to put this almost completely demolished Berlin back into operation. But what will happen if it does not succeed?

He needed another *Allional* to get through that night.

26

Lead us not into Temptation

As a Christian one must not throw away one's life on one's own authority like a dirty piece of clothing, no matter how terribly difficult life has become.

A chilly and rainy Sunday morning, the Sunday of his son's memorial service, put Api into a particularly sad and nostalgic mood. As often before, the day began with the sounds of the out-of-tune piano drifting over from a neighbouring building. Although off key, he immediately recognised the tune: it was the beautiful seventeenth-century hymn *Lobe den Herren, Praise to the Lord, the Almighty, the King of Creation*. As he listened with devotion, he thought back to the many Sunday morning coffee hours on the balcony above the roofs of Berlin. They would all be dressed in their Sunday best for the church service at 10 a.m. Then, with a smile, he remembered that not quite all of them were ready for Dieter was always the last out of bed. For a moment he lost track of time and, like his beloved son, had to hurry to ready himself for the service. Putting on his clothes, he suffered a sudden panic attack about us. His imagination painted terrible pictures of what might have happened to us. Perhaps we were not even alive any more. He had to force himself to finish dressing. By that time it was getting late and he ran into Luisenstrasse and across the street to the Charité chapel. The chapel was heavily damaged. The neo-Gothic windows were all gone and the roof with its step façade, characteristic of most Charité buildings, was partially collapsed. The weary and anxious congregation with their emaciated grey faces sat in what remained of the pews, their feet shuffling back and forth in thick layers of mortar and dust.

The service nevertheless offered Api some consolation. Pastor Küssner gave a moving sermon commemorating my uncle. He also told of our painful separation and Api's loneliness, and afterwards the congregation supported Api with their compassion. The final hymn was *Sollt ich meinem Gott nicht singen, sollt ich ihm nicht dankbar sein, Sing my soul to God who made thee*. Api gladly joined in this well-known hymn, which expresses deep faith in a God who, through everything, takes care of His children. 'When I sleep His care surrounds me, with new strength and youth imbues ...' The text was written by my grandparents' favourite hymn writer, Paul Gerhardt, often called 'the sweet singer of Lutheranism'. As he sang along with the small congregation, Api thought how Paul Gerhardt himself had lived through troubling and violent times during the seventeenth-century religious wars. He also had a strong connection with Berlin where he had served as pastor, not far from where Api was sitting just then.

I share Api's love for Paul Gerhardt, or more likely have learnt it from him. Gerhardt wrote many of the most popular Lutheran hymns, such as *Befiehl du deine Wege, Commit whatever grieves thee*, in 1656, and *O Sacred Head now Wounded*, which is sung in Lutheran churches in Germany every year during the Good Friday service. Both Api and I were particularly fond of the folksong-like evening hymn *Nun ruhen alle Wälder, Now all the woods are sleeping*. I cannot find an adequate translation for the simplicity of the verses about the closing of day, especially the fourth stanza which begins with '*Der Tag ist nun vergangen*'. My version, which I adapted from existing ones, does not ring true to my ears either, but it is the closest I can come:

> *The rule of day is over*
> *and golden stars now cover*
> *The heaven's boundless blue*

There also will I join them
when God calls me to heaven
out of this wretched earth to Him.

The service was followed by a special lunch at the clinic. Api was grateful for the rare treat but could not fully enjoy it. He had not yet completely shaken his bout of anxiety and now worried whether we had anything to eat all. But overall, this Sunday had given him back a little strength: 'I am so grateful to God and will not slacken off in my prayers to strengthen in me a true, vigorous, kindly Christianity, and a childlike trust in God's providence, and a quiet and humble submission to His will.' As if to reflect his momentary brighter mood, the rainy morning had turned into a wonderfully bright and sunny, if still cool, day.

Soon thereafter, Api found two books that became a mainstay for the rest of his time in Berlin. One was a hymnal, and the other Heinrich Spengler's *Der Kleine Pilgerstab – The Little Pilgrim's Staff –* a book of morning and evening devotions for each day of the Christian calendar year. A popular work in Germany, it had seen many editions since its first appearance in the year of Api's birth in 1888. Api's own edition, which I still have, dates from 1927. From the moment he discovered the book, he followed the *Pilgerstab*'s messages of faith, hope and love for each day. It helped him, especially since he had begun to feel that his despondency was obliterating any words of prayer he had once known. As soon as he discovered it, he fondly opened the heavy black book, noticing how the gold ornamentation on the front cover had almost disappeared under the grime, and looked up the passage for that Monday night. It came from his favourite Psalms, specifically 17, 8, and he read: 'As the apple of the eye me keep; in thy wings shade me close.'

It was from this point on in the aftermath of the war that Api clung more and more desperately to his faith to avoid a complete breakdown. He began and ended each day with a ten-minute reading from both books. He always looked forward to these morning and evening devotions, which became absolutely indispensable. Without them, he feared, he would not be able to go on. In the hymnal he preferred the section on 'Cross and Consolation', with hymns like *Ein Christ kann ohne Kreuz nicht sein, A Christian cannot live without a cross*, which reminded him that everyone had a burden to carry and that God watched over all. Every morning on waking, Api also said the little prayer with which, for more than twenty-five years, Nyussi and he had greeted each new day. It began with '*Du warst mit Deinem Schutz bei mir*', 'you were with me with your protection'. Knowing full well how familiar Nyussi was with the prayer, Api never mentioned more than the first line. However, I have not heard it before, nor have I been able to find it anywhere since.

Api always went to church on Sundays, but he hardly dared show up for services in his crumpled and dirty clothes. When Herr Max Gerhardt, his friend and former neighbour, saw Api's shabby appearance, he gave him a pair of so-called Stresemann trousers (formal, grey-striped trousers) and a black jacket to go along with them. Now it felt good to dress up on Sundays. Api also still had the single pearl tiepin that he liked to wear for festive occasions. Despite his grey hair and grey face he looked quite presentable, and less like the shabby beggar he felt he really was.

Reading about the pin, I remembered how often I had seen him with it after the war. He wore it on his tie under his white doctor's coat and, of course, always on Sundays. When I look at pictures of that time I often see him with it as well. I had forgotten all about it, but now that pearl tiepin alone can arouse happy memories of our times together.

Api divided his Sundays between the Sophien church and the Charité chapel. He chose the Sophien church when the famous Pastor Döhring was holding services there. Since 1914 Bruno Döhring, who was born in 1879 in East Prussia, had held the office of *Oberhof* and *Domprediger*, that is, Court and Cathedral Preacher, at the Cathedral of Berlin across from the royal palace at the east end of Unter den Linden. He was, of course, the last person with that title since there was no more imperial court after 1918. Döhring had been hugely popular and his cathedral had always been crowded on Sundays. When times were hard in the 1930s he had his sermons printed to be sold after the service to raise funds for the poor. After Emperor Wilhelm II was exiled to House Doorn in Holland, Döhring dispatched a copy of his sermon every week to the express train which left Berlin for Doorn so that the former emperor would have it punctually on Sunday. He continued to provide sermons until Wilhelm's death in 1941.

The cathedral was destroyed on 24 May 1944, and when both pastors at the Sophien church lost their lives in the last days of the war, Döhring helped out there and that was when Api heard his sermons. After the war, Döhring returned to his cathedral, although it remained a ruin for a long time. The cupola was not closed until 1953 and the building not restored until the 1970s, long after Döhring's death in 1961.

Pastor Döhring understood the desperate mood of his congregation and designed each sermon for the needs of the people and the times. He knew that many had no place to stay; that they lived huddled among the ruins in terror and insecurity, ravaged by hunger and sickness, with little hope for the future. The number of suicides increased daily. Pastor Döhring may well have known, as did Api, that in Berlin-Neukölln the gas which had just been turned on had to be shut off again because too many used it to kill themselves. Doctors also knew that at least half their patients did not come to be cured but asked for poisons to kill themselves.

Api often reported the gist of Döhring's sermon in his diary. On Sunday 3 June, for instance, Pastor Döhring tried to assure the sad congregation that God would not forget the poor and that the hope of miserable people lasted for eternity. Although these words did him good, Api's thoughts strayed to the old church in Suderburg and he hoped God would forgive him this inattentiveness. His mind came back to the sermon just in time to hear Pastor Döhring's warning, which was so fitting for himself and for many of the desperate people around him: 'As a Christian one must not throw away one's life on one's own authority like a dirty piece of clothing, no matter how terribly difficult life has become. God will not forget about His poor people.' Api felt as if Pastor Döhring was talking to him personally and he fervently prayed that his faith in God's loving guidance would strengthen him to bear anything that was to come.

On another Sunday Api recollected the pastor speaking about how with Christ, and in Christ, all paths were possible which God had ordained for us. Api paid close attention and later quoted parts of the sermon in his diary. Döhring had said:

These days in particular will show that the mature Christian stands infinitely richer and firmer, and of an iron will – even if he has to sacrifice everything including himself – than someone who has not allowed himself to be touched by God. We cannot comprehend Him if he has not touched us. The longing for God is fulfilled only if someone says: 'I cannot live without my God.' But with Him we can bear everything and we must continue to live until He says 'It is enough now'. We should not urge the fulfilment of our wishes, however justified they may be. But we must wait, wait with faith in God and the sincerest love of our Lord Jesus Christ. 'No one comes to the Father but through me.'

At the Charité chapel, Api heard much the same message. Pastor Küssner, likewise, was warning against the temptation of suicide and held out the hope that a strong faith would protect one from such a step. 'Lead us not into temptation, but deliver us of all evil' was his theme. Like Pastor Döhring, he was well aware that many in his congregation, Api included, were contemplating suicide as a last escape from their hopeless situation.

27

The Silence

I have not found a single German ready to admit his
personal guilt in the war.

S itting by his window on the evening of Tuesday 29 May, Api drew
out the slim pencil attached in a loop to the diary and began to write
about a topic most painful to him: his *Pg* status and the question of
guilt. He reflected that he had often spoken out 'with my patients
and other officers with an openness which certainly could have had fateful
consequences for me'. Then addressing Nyussi he added: 'You know how I
and all of us have condemned those shameful measures of the Nazis.' As to
taking action, 'who could have done anything against this and how??' Yet at
the same time he also voiced regret that he had been unable to do anything.
In the end he felt that just being a member of the Party should not make him
liable to persecution and punishment. It was a distressing subject for Api
and he revisited it only briefly on other occasions in his diary. The following
day he still thought about these issues when he wrote a sort of farewell to
us: 'Should we not see each other again: thanks be to God for lovely days
and that we never wanted evil for anyone or went past anyone's suffering
without compassion.'

Reading this today, I am confused on many levels. I understand that
once Api had joined the Party, he was caught, unable to do anything but

complain, and even then only in secret. And that, therefore, he now felt unjustly condemned in the rush to punish all former members of the Party indiscriminately. I also am reassured by his compassion for the suffering of others, which I have experienced first hand. What bewilders me is that Api seems to talk of the war but does not mention the persecution of the Jews and the concentration camps, either here or elsewhere in his diary. He may not have known details about the concentration camps at the time when they occurred, many Germans did not. Even the well-connected journalist Ursula von Kardoff only found out after the war about the mass murder of Jews. But Api had surely witnessed many instances of persecution, had seen how Jewish businesses were destroyed, Jewish doctors disappeared and even how Jewish children suddenly were absent from the schools my mother and uncle attended. I wonder whether 'those shameful measures of the Nazis' was a reference, albeit inadequate and oblique, to the Holocaust?

Whatever he did not know during the war, by the end of May 1945, when Api was writing this, news about the horrors of the death camps had been made widely public by the Allies in reports, films, news releases, posters and over the radio. I remember when I was just 3 years old that in the small village of Suderburg I picked up the word *KZ*, short for concentration camp, because I heard it mentioned everywhere. I knew it was important to the grown ups since they were always talking about it, but I had no idea what it meant. So one day I was singing '*KZ, KZ*' to myself when my mother rushed up and told me not to say that. I stopped. But I still did not know what was wrong since everyone else used that word all the time.

So why did Api say nothing? This is particularly striking when he himself suffered from persecution as a *Pg*, and feared arrest at any time. He was prepared to leave at a moment's notice in the middle of the night, his clothes always ready for immediate departure. Yet nowhere did he see his fate in relation to that of millions of Jews during the Nazi terror. Does his silence imply that he was in any way in agreement with the racism that ended up costing millions of lives? Is silence itself a sign of guilt? I cannot square this with his ethical, tolerant and compassionate world view. One small, if inconclusive, corroboration is a letter from a Jewish colleague I found among Api's papers. I know nothing of the circumstances, only that the writer told Api that he had escaped from the Charité to Brazil from where he was writing. He wrote how much Api's friendship had meant to him and that, except for him and some members of his own family still left in Berlin, he cared for no one there.

Perhaps Api said nothing because he felt that it was too terrible to dwell on at a time when his nerves were overwrought with fear and desolation? Perhaps he was too ashamed? Or did he hide his head in the sand? What could he have done then and what could he say as he was writing his diary? Who could have imagined atrocities of a kind and on a scale as were perpetrated by the Nazis? What collective guilt do the German people bear? Would I have acted any differently? Despite all these unanswered questions I simply cannot imagine that Api condoned fanatical hate and a desire to persecute others.

Nevertheless, this silence still troubles and bewilders me, although I have learned since that Api shared this trait with most people at that time. Even today, most Germans of his generation and even the next are reluctant to speak about the Nazi persecution of the Jews. In fact, it is not even my generation but the one after me that is breaking through the silence. Many books are just beginning to come out in twenty-first-century Germany that refer to silence in the title, such as *Silent Perpetrators, Talking Grandchildren* (2006), *Silence Hurts* (2008) and *After a Long Silence* (2000), to name but a few. Just recently, in 2009, I happened to speak on the phone with a man from a village in Germany. His family lived next door to Kurt Simon, whose biography I had just finished. Kurt had immigrated to the United States and today, in his nineties, he sees it as his greatest life achievement to have rescued his parents out of Germany in 1937, although much of the rest of his family perished in the Holocaust. The man I talked to on the phone probably is in his forties, so he was born well after the war. He admitted that his village has not yet come to terms with the Nazi period and the persecution of the few Jews who had lived there. 'The old people here,' he said, 'still refuse to speak about the Nazis and the persecution of the Jews.'

Immediately after the end of the war, the Allies interpreted this German silence as a crass evasion of responsibility. 'I have not found a single German ready to admit his personal guilt in the war,' reported war correspondent Alan Moorehead. This assessment, however, appears too simplistic an interpretation of what Germans felt at that time. Moorehead's view can be explained by the shock and the horror he and the world at large felt as the truth about the death camps became known and images of mass graves, gas chambers and skeletal survivors appeared on newsreels. But it does not, and perhaps cannot, be expected to offer a nuanced insight into the minds and hearts of Germans in 1945, who at that point were themselves struggling to survive.

One evening, after a meal of peas and bits of meat that smelled bad, Api sought refuge from his worries in a contemplation of nature. Despite the smoke clouds, which still drifted across the peaceful evening sky, and despite the vista of charred rafters and ruins, he wrote:

> it is once again an evening of rare May beauty. Not a breeze stirs under the faintly blue shimmering sky, and a few pink evening clouds hang in the mother of pearl blue, almost motionless and transparently delicate like spirits of a goodness and nobility that has vanished from the earth. And as always a few swifts chase each other through this sublime stillness in a last joyful game. On many such evenings our four leaf clover sat on our little unforgettably cosy balcony, full of thoughts of peace, and in conversation about human ethics and divine providence! No one suspected anything about the brewing calamity until our leaders left the paths of lawfulness and we – well knowing but impotent – had to watch how the little boat drifted.

I am not surprised by the nostalgia Api voiced here, but I cannot understand his naivety. Or is it a deliberate blindness? I am not sure what time Api is talking about when he says that they did not suspect anything, or at what point he thought that the Nazis left the paths of lawfulness whilst he was 'well knowing but impotent'. This passage is one of those moments when I would love to talk with Api and ask him what he meant, although I am not sure I would have done it anyway. It is also an occasion when retracing Api's steps becomes most problematic for me.

28

Suicidal Thoughts

I relive this nightmare every day, and cannot endure
it any longer.

For Api, as no doubt for most Berliners, the first month after the end
of the war had brought no peace. But at the end of May he saw just
a small ray of hope when the first patient showed up. Api was glad
that he had risked the investment in new instruments. The next
day he even had two patients, but he knew that it was far too early to count
on an ever-increasing number finding their way to his door. One of them
told him yet another disquietening rumour. The man said that everyone
who had been evacuated during the war now had to return to Berlin. After
he was gone, Api kept thinking about this: 'Shall I wish for it, shall I not wish
for it?? People are allowed to take with them only what they can carry on
foot, and bread (only bread) for five days. My God, you poorest ones, and
without my help!'

Whenever he could get away from helping at the North Sanatorium,
Api busied himself in his surgery. Patients continued to straggle in, and
occasionally a Russian officer was among them. Api thought that even in
the days of his earliest beginnings he had not experienced such long hours
of fruitless waiting. He consoled himself with the thought that without
public transport it was difficult for patients to reach him. But every time

he imagined that he heard a movement by his door, he jumped up with a pounding heart. If it was indeed a patient, he would have liked to embrace him, so glad was he to see someone looking for his services. Most often, however, there was no one there, just his wishful imagination playing tricks on him. Nevertheless, every time a gust of wind moved the loose floorboards of the waiting room, he was there at the door ready to receive his patient.

Seeing his surgery open, Fräulein Herzog, his former nurse assistant, stopped by and they agreed to work together again, even if there was not much to do. She had, she said, nowhere else to go. Her life was desperate, although I can catch only glimpses of the details in the diary. Already middle aged, Fräulein Herzog was struggling with the loss of most of her family and trying to survive by herself in Berlin. She was a brave and resourceful woman, but there were times when she just collapsed. Api mentioned one such incident when Fräulein Herzog burst into his surgery, desperate and in tears. She told him between sobs: 'I cannot go on. The only solution I see is to kill myself.' Api, who had experienced similar depressions himself all too often, sat down to talk with her for several hours.

Fräulein Herzog told him that they had been a poor family but they had been happy together and now all that was gone. Her 12-year-old brother had been taken away by the SS and she had not heard from him since. Then she had watched her sister die in an explosion. Between sobs, Fräulein Herzog explained what had happened. The two of them had been caught in a narrow passage between two streets near their lodgings when an incendiary bomb exploded. Somehow Fräulein Herzog managed to get away. She immediately turned back to look for her sister; however, the passage was blocked with screaming people. Then a fireman grabbed her, refusing to let her pass. Without being able to do anything, she had to watch the flames and listen to the screams of people, including her sister, caught in the conflagration. Fräulein Herzog cried: 'I relive this nightmare every day, and cannot endure it any longer.'

Api was at a loss of how to console her except to tell her how his faith in God had got him through his most desperate hours. He knew there was little he could say in response to such heartbreak, but just hearing another voice and feeling another's care might do some good. Gradually, Fräulein

Herzog grew calmer. Her courage, which had not let her down often, slowly returned and she said, wiping away the last of her tears, that she was determined once again to continue the struggle, whatever it might bring.

Fräulein Herzog was by no means alone in her suicidal thoughts. Every day Api heard about friends and acquaintances who could not bear the strain of anxiety and hopelessness and killed themselves. Api mentioned only those among them who were from their neighbourhood and whom Nyussi would also have known. The wife of pharmacist Dr Weinreich, Frau Ludwig and her daughter and Butcher Boemer who shot himself were the most recent fatalities. Even one of the patients at the North Sanatorium had hanged himself. There had already been so many suicides: women who had suffered rape, men who could not bear the uncertainty and terror, entire families who saw no way out.

29

Professional Development

I have to think backwards again and again, one can't
look ahead yet.

To prepare himself for the resumption of his career, Api studied
textbooks on ophthalmology. Whenever he had energy enough
after his day's work and the light was still good in his attic – for
he still was without electricity – he sat down to educate himself
further in his field. In this respect he saw one advantage of being on
Moscow time: it stayed light until well after 10 p.m. He feared that he had
lost much expertise during his military service in the war years and needed
to prepare himself again for his career as eye surgeon. But he did not even
know whether, as a *Pg*, he would be allowed to open a practice. He hoped
that what a doctor friend had heard in the mayor's office was true, that
simply paying a membership without activity, which was Api's case, would
not be a reason against it. Stuck in the Russian occupation zone, Api was
caught in repetitive cycles of minor ups and, increasingly, major downs.
Small bits of progress with his surgery were easily upset by sickness, doubt
and despair of getting free of Berlin. So he took refuge in picturing the
happy past: 'I have to think backwards again and again, one can't look
ahead yet.'

As he was checking the back of his desk in his surgery, Api uncovered a little picture album. Thumbing through it brought back the happy times associated with them and he broke down in bleak hopelessness. I still have that tiny brown album and can see what Api looked at that day. It is only large enough for one small picture on each page. Its pretty, marbled cover decorated with a faded red stripe at the binding is undamaged, a survivor from the past. I flip through the pages and see a record of my grandparents' early days on Luisenstrasse in the 1920s. There is my mother's first day of school on Albrechtstrasse, which Mike and I later visited. The picture shows her in knee socks, a short pleated skirt and a sailor's top with stripes at the neck and wrists. These must have been fashionable at the time, but over twenty years later I remember also having just such a sailor outfit for special occasions. I have very similar pictures of me in my blue-and-white striped sailor's top at the same age my mother was in the album. She is clutching her *Schultüte*, the large colourful paper cone stuffed with sweets first-graders get from their parents to help ease them into the beginning of school. One can see that she is at once proud to go to school and afraid of this new world into which she is about to step.

On another page I see Nyussi, her long dark hair gathered at the neck, in a slim skirt and round-necked patterned blouse. She is leaning against Api on their balcony. It must have been a weekend for he is dressed in his leisure-time vest and knickerbockers and holding a paper on his knee. Next there is Nyussi again, this time in a cape and dark hat pulled over her eyes. She stands in front of their building with my mother crouching beside her, a big bow on her head, and my chubby, curly headed Uncle Dieter at her other side. The next picture, obviously taken at the same time, shows Nyussi sitting on a bench with Api, who is formally dressed in a three-piece suit with high-collared shirt, tie and bowler hat, holding an umbrella. Nyussi's cape is open this time, revealing a startlingly light dress, which has a flowing scarf at the neck.

In the middle of the album I come across one picture of myself, which must have been added later. It was taken in Bevensen, where we had moved from the Suderburg cottage. I am 8 years old, standing in the bedroom I still shared with my grandparents and bending over a pram of which I was very proud. The Hinzpeter painting of the Chiemsee is hanging over the double bed, and I notice that I am wearing just as big a bow on my head as my mother was when she was my age. I wonder who stuck this picture into the little album. Flipping through the pages once again, the album strikes me, as it must have Api, as from another world than the one in which he found himself in 1945.

June began with an order that bewildered Api, as it did all Berliners. It was one of those absurd occurrences that happen in times of chaos, especially since there were four nations trying to govern Germany. On 1 June an order went out that every house that still was inhabited must fly the Russian, American, English and French national flags in a size of at least 85cm x 180cm, which is about 2.5ft x 6ft. No one knew why this had to be done or how to accomplish it all of a sudden. Those who still had Nazi flags hidden away quickly cut out the red part for the Russian flag. Everyone looked for bits of red, white and blue cloth to stitch together makeshift flags to hang out the windows. As they set about this task there was consternation among Berliners about how many stars to put in the American flag. So, always quick witted, they added a line to the popular German children's song:

> *Weisst du wieviel Sternlein stehen?*
> Do you know how many stars are in the sky?
> *Denn du musst sie schleunigst nähen.*
> For you have to sew them now.

One major topic at the North Sanatorium was that the Russian occupation administration had decreed that, for every Russian who was shot by members of Operation Werwolf, fifty members of the Nazi Party would be executed. Operation Werwolf had been the Nazis' last-ditch effort at resistance; a clandestine force that was supposed to wage guerrilla warfare on the occupiers and sabotage their installations. It never amounted to much, but all four Allies took the threat seriously, believing that Werwolf activities could 'hardly be overrated'. Their fierce measures against the population in the early days of the occupation can in part be attributed to this fear of Werwolf attacks. Api saw no evidence of any Werwolf activity; indeed he never believed in the operation, regarding it as another terrible legacy of the Nazis, 'this gang of criminals'.

Early in June an unexpected treasure arrived in his surgery, a beautiful Siemens radio. It belonged to his friend Herr Gerhardt, a former fellow lodger at Luisenstrasse 41, who was hoping to join Api in the apartment when it was ready. Api hoped that the radio would provide better news than the rumour mill, and he was eager to hear more than gossip about the seemingly endless numbers of new orders and regulations from the Soviets. He carefully placed it on his little table and admired the shiny wooden box. It had a brown fabric front with metallic threads woven in. There were two large black dials, one for switching on and the other for choosing a station.

Api turned the dial, hoping for a news broadcast or at least some classical music. But he found only the throbbing rhythms of dance music: 'I cannot listen and do not want to. Dance music in this misery is perverse, paradoxical for my tortured longing heart. Nevertheless one has to listen in hope of any news and to find out about the constant stream of new regulations.' Of particular interest to him were any clues as to whether evacuees were to come back to Berlin or whether Berliners could leave the city. So he kept the radio on anyway.

Professionally, Api had some good news. Starting on 4 June, Professor Löhlein invited him to collaborate in his eye surgery class at the university. The professor was in the process of setting up a class to be held each morning from 8 a.m. to 11 a.m. In early May Api had worked under Professor Löhlein at the military hospital on Ziegelstrasse. He was delighted at this opportunity to assist in the class and relieved, too, that he had taken up his theoretical readings again.

To make himself more presentable for his new assignment, Api went in search of a haircut. He found a barber on the ground floor of a roofless building. As he sat in the barber's chair to be shorn, he had leisure to study himself in the mirror. He was shocked at the image that stared back at him. How much he had changed! The last weeks had turned him into an aged, run-down and lifeless old man. His face was as grey as his surroundings in this dust-covered ruin of a city. His once clear and usually smiling blue eyes looked too large for his emaciated face and they stared back at him without light. Deep lines ran from his nose to his thin mouth, and the little laugh lines by his eyes had become invisible in his ashen face. But if only, he thought as he studied himself, if only he could see a clear road ahead, how gladly would he work and what strength he could still muster to support us and make a new start! That happy vision, however, was still only a dream.

The fulfilment of this dream was further threatened when Api developed intestinal problems, which steadily got worse. He was afraid of an attack of dysentery such as he had suffered at the beginning of the First World War and which had had such fearful consequences. Some mornings his stomach cramps and diarrhoea got so bad that he was afraid of passing out. He knew that dysentery was becoming widespread. Since he had hardly any eye patients and the need for doctors was so great, Api often functioned as a general practitioner making house calls and helping people in distress. For the most part he did not charge for his services, for many of his patients were worse off than he was himself.

30

Nyussi's Birthday

*I could, I would, I should shoulder my packed
rucksack and come to you without hesitation, and
without doubting my strength to master the distance!*

The early days of June brought another trial for Api's already
overwrought nerves: 9 June was Nyussi's birthday. At the
beginning of the month he had started a letter to her to which
he added every day. He had little hope of this ever-growing letter
reaching her, as indeed it did not, but the very act of writing helped him.
In the process he remembered the many birthdays they had spent together;
the early happy ones and the sad ones of the war. He gave them names:
the first Dahlem birthday in 1920 with his mother's flowers; the Buick
birthday when they had bought their first big car, the 'green one', in 1926;
the rose bouquet birthday on holiday in Bad Elster in 1943 when, on that
very day, they heard for certain that my father had died; and 1944, just a
year ago, the bouquet of tiny wood flowers with the paltry little cake at the
Joachimsthal birthday where Nyussi, my mother and I stayed briefly after
we were bombed out.

Api began Nyussi's birthday, Saturday 9 June, by opening his book of
daily devotions to that day, the first Saturday after Trinitatis. What he
found seemed to be addressed to him directly: 'Then he said to them: "You

of little faith, why are you so anxious?"' The commentary that followed these words from Matthew 8, 26, sounded equally applicable to him. It said that as long as Jesus is in our house and in our hearts, there can be no ruin and no undoing. Api tried to internalise these words of consolation. Then, since Nyussi was unreachable, he picked up her sweater and kissed it instead. He was well aware that this was going too far, but it was a defence strategy that helped him to endure his isolation and assuage his fears a little. He wrote:

> Sometimes I have such a terrible worry about you. I have worn your little woollen jacket once more today since it was chilly in the morning and have – kissed it fervently. I know that this almost no longer is adoring love but rather a cult. But where shall I go with my sometimes really overpowering longings for you all!

Before church the following morning, Api took a few moments to study the sky from his attic window:

> A sky full of peace and infinity in which a few delicate feather clouds drift silently together with an early swallow. Otherwise a nameless stillness and devotion in God's wonderful nature which will also lift my eyes and heart above the ruins and the sorrows of this poor earth.

Church music from a radio across the street drifted up to him and he thought that perhaps his faith was growing firmer:

> I am getting a little closer to a Christianity that finds a strong hold in its love for Jesus and God, and in its faith in their loving guidance. One has to learn to pray. First comes the joy in prayer and then the strength and the capacity to draw real powerful consolation from this search for God and the feeling of His nearness!

Even his faith could not lessen his yearning, however: 'I could, I would, I should shoulder my packed rucksack and come to you without hesitation, and without doubting my strength to master the distance!'

Api did have one way of celebrating the day after Nyussi's birthday. He had been given a ticket for a musical matinee at the Deutsches Theatre. The Russian occupation forces were trying to provide the population with a respite from hunger and fear by supporting concerts, theatre and even opera performances. These had begun as early as May 1945, but this was Api's first such occasion. He had not been sure that he would be able to attend because of his continuing stomach problems. However, not wanting to miss such an opportunity, he forced himself to get ready.

From 1905 to 1930 the Deutsches Theatre had been managed by Max Reinhardt, who had also given the building its present look by adding a neo-classical front. How many hours Nyussi and he had spent there enjoying the classical German repertoire, as well as modern plays by Bernard Shaw, Gerhart Hauptmann and many others. Most of the great German actors of the time had appeared there, among them Paula Wessely, Kaethe Dorsch, Ewald Balser and Gustav Gründgens. As soon as Api and Nyussi could afford it, they had bought a yearly subscription to the theatre for all four of them.

When Api turned into Schumannstrasse, he saw the Deutsches Theatre like an oasis in the devastation all around. It had remained almost completely unharmed. Api stood outside the theatre for a long time gazing at the white columns of its familiar façade, which was set back from the street in a quiet little square. When he walked inside he saw that it, too, looked much the same as he had known it. He greeted the half-round auditorium with its gilded columns like an old friend and was overcome by memories of their visits in the unrecoverable past. The hall, decorated in white, gold and red as of old, had a festive and yet cosy atmosphere. Api did not mention what pieces he heard that afternoon, only that the music soothed him. Music always had a powerful effect on him. It made him feel connected to suffering humanity and less alone.

31

Walking through a Nightmare

I can only entrust these happy images to this little book without life or purpose or use ... But, for me it is an irreplaceably beautiful substitute for the community with you which I miss so painfully, one of my dearest hours in the day!!

Whenever he went out, Api saw so many who were far worse off than he was. Berlin was choked with refugees. Streams of ragged people from the eastern parts of Germany who had fled before the Russians were limping and crawling about in the centre of Berlin. They carried old suitcases or dragged their few belongings in carts and wheelbarrows through the streets. He saw old men and women who could hardly walk any more, and others who used their last strength to hold their babies in their arms. Compared with such misery, he had to count himself lucky. About 3 million refugees came through Berlin in those days.

One day Api noticed an old tubercular woman lying in the gutter. She could not go on for weakness and just lay there coughing but otherwise apathetic. He went to her and tried to make her more comfortable, but she did not respond. He offered her a piece of bread he had brought along, the pasty black bread so despised by the Russian officer, which was all he had. She just left it lying there. He could do nothing more for her. The hospitals were overcrowded and there were so many like her in the streets of Berlin:

> the still never ending columns of refugees who, with their last strength and together with 4–5 year old children, drag, panting, two or four wheeled carts containing the beggar's remains of their possessions in order to reach any kind of shelter before the curfew, or at least come a little closer to an often imaginary destination!

The image of that old woman stayed with him throughout the day.

Injured soldiers, armless and legless, who moved on old margarine cartons put on wheels were another common sight. I still remember in the early 1950s such war veterans coming to our door offering pictures, usually greeting cards of landscapes or flowers, 'painted with the foot' or 'painted with the mouth'. We always gave them money and food and I was amazed at how delicate and detailed the pictures were.

Api knew that epidemics were almost inevitable without sanitation, rubbish pickups or even proper removal of the dead. As the weather grew warmer, a plague of vermin, lice, flies, maggots and rats infested the city. Luckily, rats did not make it up to Api's attic room above the North Sanatorium, but flies swarmed in black clouds; bluebottles as large as he had only seen them when he was a young military doctor in Macedonia during the First World War. Without window panes, it was impossible to keep them out. He slew at least fifty each evening before going to bed, and yet swarms still buzzed around him throughout the night.

Weakened by sickness, Api tried to spend ever more time on his silent communion with us and God. He made sure that he had a few moments each day 'to dream into the evening sky' thinking of us and of the past. He sought consolation in the idea that if all else failed him and he would not see us again, he was left at the last with his faith that 'we were all united in God and that we would be granted a blessed reunion in His kingdom where there was no separation, no worry, no anxiety, no misery'. Yet he did not entirely give up hope, writing to us:

161

My dearest, evening has come again, another day is gone, and the heart that does not want to, and cannot, unlearn hope rejoices to have come one little step closer perhaps to the goal always floating before it, our reunion in a world at peace.

Api's intestinal problems worsened and the charcoal tablets he took did not help much. Charcoal was a popular remedy against diarrhoea. As a small child in Suderburg, when I had a bout of diarrhoea, my mother would give me charcoal tablets out of a little metal tin. I did not mind their chalky taste and delighted in the way they turned my mouth black.

Api's 'down' mood – he used the English word – was made worse by a desolate day in his surgery. Not a single patient showed up, perhaps because Berlin was being pelted by severe rainstorms and hurricane-like gusts of wind. As Api walked back to the attic after his fruitless day, he had to take cover many times because walls and roofs of damaged buildings crumbled under the storm, and shingles rained down on the pavement. At one point his path was blocked because an entire house had collapsed in front of him. And the trials of that day were not over yet. Three Russians suddenly appeared out of the ruins and threatened to arrest him. Shaking with sickness and fear, Api produced his medical papers and the soldiers let him go. That night, Api thought that sleeping pills would not be enough and he took opium. It was the first and only time during these months that he had recourse to opium. I know nothing about the medicinal use of opium at that time, but his access to medication certainly was an advantage Api had over the general population.

Despite feeling weak himself Api continued his visits to the sick. He earned a little money but he also wanted to assist as many people as he could. At the same time, he hoped that perhaps the contacts he made would help build his own practice in the future. With that aim in mind he also went to see general practitioners, asking them to refer eye patients to him. These visits were particularly hard for him. Although he tried to disguise them with all kinds of tricks and pretences, he felt everyone knew that he was begging and his pride suffered badly.

To help him recover from his stomach problem, the always generous Herr Gerhardt made him a present of a bottle of burgundy. Api's first instinct was to save the rare treat, to *knausern*, be stingy, once again as was his habit.

But then he thought about how his son had often scolded him for being too parsimonious and not enjoying something when the occasion arose. So hearing his dear Dieter say to him, 'Dad, don't be such a skinflint', he treated himself to a glass.

Wednesday 13 June brought a major improvement in the attic when electricity was reconnected. For the first time he could write his diary by electric light. This also meant that he could read his medical texts well into the night. It gave him a little sense that, perhaps, a normal life would be possible again. The very next day a glazier appeared and replaced the cardboard of his windows with glass. This helped to keep the flies at bay. Then, on Friday 15 June, Api suffered a particularly severe intestinal attack. Again he was terrified of coming down with dysentery, remembering his illness in 1914 and its awful, long-lasting consequences. For the first time he stayed in bed until ten in the morning, but then he felt compelled to get up and make his way laboriously to his practice. It turned out to be a trip made in vain since no one came. He sat idly in his office, unable to read or do anything productive. This in itself was a burden to a man who hated vacuity and felt one always had to do something useful and constructive. Api was totally discouraged.

Having had nothing to eat and feeling particularly faint, the walk back made a surreal impression on him and he suffered what I now think of as a panic attack. It seemed as if the shockingly blue sky was laughing at him and at the grey burnt-out ruins he passed. By contrast, the black window holes glared at him ominously in their deadness. He saw himself as if from a great distance almost swallowed up by rubble and stones. Api was walking through a nightmare from which there was no awakening. When he got to his building, he had to rest often to climb the four sets of stairs to the attic; he was bathed in sweat from the effort. Once safely in his 'swallow's nest', the familiar surroundings helped him to calm down.

Sitting by the window, he tried to recover from the living nightmare he had experienced on his way home, which seemed even worse than the recurring nightmares of his dreams. At times he feared that he could not tell horrible dreams from reality. To counteract these images and still his pounding heart, he concentrated his mind on picturing a reunion with us. He visualised himself walking down the streets of Suderburg and knocking on our cottage window as he had done in what now seemed like an age ago, but was only a few months. He dwelled on the happy reunion in the most vivid colours; on the joy in our eyes; on holding me in his arms; on how we would sit down to a simple meal and then walk together on the sandy path outside the farmhouse with a view of the Blue Mountain.

Then his imagination switched to paint another scene. We had all come back to Berlin. The old apartment, so steeped in happiness and sorrow, had been restored, his practice was picking up and we all lived together in peace and security. He imagined his Hinzpeter painting on the wall of their home. It depicted Alpine woods which he loved so much. He remembered how, long ago when he had been ill, Nyussi had taken the picture off its hook in the living room and put it in his bedroom so that he could enjoy it. She hoped that looking at the forest scene, so similar to their hiking excursions, would help him recover. Then he thought of that small oil painting that Nyussi had taken to Suderburg. It had been a surprise gift from the artist because Api had treated him for free. The painting showed Saint Martin cutting his cloak in half to share with a naked beggar. I remember it well for it was one of the pieces we rescued out of Berlin in 1945 and it held a place of honour wherever we lived. On her last trip to Vienna my mother brought it back with her to her home in Champaign, Illinois. Whenever I visit my stepfather, I study the stark picture, the wintry landscape covered in bleak snow, the back of the spectral naked beggar in the foreground and Saint Martin bending down toward him from his horse while cutting his cloak with his sword. My eyes invariably are drawn to the dark-red cloak, which provides the only splotch of colour in an otherwise grim scene of browns, whites and greys. As we looked at the picture together, Api was fond of telling me the story of Saint Martin, who had been a Roman soldier but converted to become a monk and led a simple life dedicated to helping others.

Just by focusing on such dreams, Api felt himself grow strong in his goal of taking care of us. To be able to work for us as a free man without the perpetual worry about personal security for himself and us – that alone could restore him. However, coming back to reality, all he could do was:

> entrust these happy images to this little book without life or purpose when I don't even know whether you will ever read it. But for me it is a substitute for the community with you which I miss so painfully, one of my dearest hours in the day!!

32

Living in Insecurity

The German people behave in such a manner among themselves that Russian commandants already have imprisoned denunciators with open expressions of scorn for such a spirit between them.

I n the latter part of June, Api's physical condition improved and he was relieved that he had escaped the worst without succumbing to dysentery. He could take a few more spoonfuls of the flour or semolina soup, which is all he had but which he had not been able to keep down before. As soon as he felt better, Api, as always, made plans. Since he had been lucky to get the loan of a bike, he would ride to RL 101, the Westend Hospital, to see about the dining room set he had left in storage there after the bombing of 1943. Api was allowed to do this because of his connections to the Westend Hospital, especially Department 17, the large eye station. Perhaps, he mused, he could install the dining room in Luisenstrasse so that there would be some furniture ready for us? On his way to the North Sanatorium he thought about using his free time next Saturday to cycle to the Westend Hospital and check whether his furniture was still there.

First, however, he had to report once again to the Health Department. He was never given more than an hour's notice of these meetings. The Russians were concerned about the rise of dysentery and wanted the input of doctors in an effort to avoid a worse epidemic. Api always wondered what could be done when patients could not be isolated and there were insufficient medications, no rubbish pickups, hardly any window panes to keep out the flies, no water pipes and no flushing toilets. How were they to avoid an epidemic under such conditions?

When Api had made it back to his attic, he even felt a little hungry. He had his first full meal after his illness and accompanied it with another glass of the burgundy. He ate some peas and potatoes but left the meat because it smelled so bad. He had taught himself to eat meat for the calories, no matter in what condition, but with his stomach still shaky he did not want to risk it. It was so difficult to catch up after an illness. For the first time Api mentioned that he had a newspaper to read with his meal. Although papers had appeared for weeks already, Api may not have been able to get hold of a copy until now, or perhaps he had not wanted to read papers since they offered nothing but the Soviet perspective and he never had been an eager newspaper reader anyway. Amazingly, through the bombing and the occupation, Berlin had been only fifteen days without any newspaper.

Newspapers had always flourished in the city. At their height in 1928, Berlin had had exactly 100 daily newspapers and many more weekly ones. The Nazis, of course, forbade and censored most of them, wanting only their own voice heard. The first post-war edition in Berlin was the *Tägliche Rundschau, The Daily Overview*, which appeared on 15 May. It was put out by the Russians and contained mainly articles translated from *Pravda* that talked about German war crimes and the efforts of the Soviet people to rebuild their country devastated by the German army. Day by day the news reports continued in this vein. The front page of the *Tägliche Rundschau* on 9 June, for example, carried headlines such as 'Life Reawakens out of the Ruins' and 'The Soviet Union heals the Wounds of the War'. These articles did not deal with Berlin or Germany, but focused on the Soviet Union and its struggle to recover. They stressed that the Soviet Union had conquered Germany in the field, and now was fighting a second war to undo the damage done by the Germans. 'The peoples of the Soviet Union rightfully will remember that this devastation is the work of the Germans. Its complete restitution is Germany's duty.' Another article boasted of the progress that had already been made. Before the war. Ukrainian coal mines, destroyed by the German army, had produced on average 3,200 tons of coal a month. Now with new equipment they produced 6,000 tons. The only news about Germany itself on this front page concerned the suicide of a former *Gauleiter*, a district commander, and the arrest of a man who had been in charge of a concentration camp. Yet the paper claimed that it was the '*Frontzeitung für die deutsche Bevölkerung*', 'The Front Paper for the German Population'.

The next day, Monday 18 June, General Bersarin died in a motorcycle accident. He was only 41 years old. The people of Berlin mourned his death. They had loved the youthful dark-haired general with his passion for motorcycles and cheered when they saw him speeding past them. Api shared the general feeling and noted that Bersarin had been 'energetic and apparently just. A shame.'

On Thursday 21 June Api at last found opportunity to make that trip to the Westend Hospital to check up on his dining room furniture. He felt invigorated as he began to pedal the 8km to his destination and grateful to his friend for having loaned him the bike. The ride took him straight west from Luisenstrasse and in his mind it seemed as if, with each turn of the wheel, he was coming a little closer to us. He even figured out that after having gone both ways he would have covered one-fifteenth of the trip to Suderburg. With a bike like the one he now rode, it could be possible. It was a beautiful fresh morning and the physical activity cheered him. He cycled along the East–West Axis to the Victory Column, the avenue which was to be part of Hitler's plan for his 'World Capital Germania'. But the stink of corpses drifted over from the Landwehr Canal, tree trunks stuck out from heaps of ruins, and weeds and even trees had begun to grow on the rubble. Immeasurable columns of pedestrians trudged through this wasteland, from the Knie, where Api had had to seek cover a few weeks ago, across the devastated Tiergarten to the Brandenburg Gate. Many of them had to walk an hour and a half to work each day and then back the same distance at night. As the road to the Westend Hospital still stretched out before him, Api was glad that he had set out so early for it soon became very hot. His attic, which had been chilly at the end of May, now had turned almost unbearably warm.

Api reached the Westend Hospital at ten in the morning. He headed straight for the storage room where he found his dining room pieces just as he had left them. Since most of his other furniture had been destroyed, this beautiful undamaged set of shiny walnut furniture was a huge joy for him. In his delight he scheduled its delivery to Luisenstrasse immediately. However, as soon as he had made the arrangements with the movers, he regretted it: 'Wouldn't everything be safer where it was?' He planned to cancel the order right away. This episode was further indication of his indecisiveness and he was once more depressed by his weakness to make any decision even about matters which earlier would have been trivial for him. This constant back and forth alone was enough to wear him out.

It was early afternoon when he arrived back in his Luisenstrasse surgery where another pleasant surprise awaited him. A nice bunch of patients was there to greet him. Among them was Frau Grossmann, an acquaintance who was to help him much in the next weeks. She told him that the middle-class suburbs of Friedenau and Steglitz, immediately south of the Tiergarten, had been spared almost completely; houses were intact and businesses open as in peacetime. And, she added excited about bringing such good news, there was only one eye doctor in the area. As she was telling him this, Api thought fleetingly that Friedenau had been the very first place he had considered back in 1924 when he had wanted to start his own practice. Then he heard Frau Grossmann, who herself lived at Riemenschneiderweg 40 in Friedenau, give this advice: 'Why don't you move there. It would be a much better place to start a practice than in this heap of ruins.'

This suggestion, kindly meant, threw Api into a new quandary. Would he get permission for a change of location? And, more importantly to his always grateful and sentimental mind, how could he give up his place of work so dear to him, which had supported them all so well over the years? Seeing his hesitation, Frau Grossmann repeated her suggestion and even offered to talk to the local mayor. But Api just did not know what to do and saw problems and obstacles everywhere. One major hurdle was that he would have to get permission to move from the Russian to the American zone and he did not want to attract the attention of the Russian administration.

Api thought all evening about the possibility of moving. In addition to Frau Grossmann's idea of Friedenau, his colleague, Dr Hüdepohl, had suggested that he apply to Hedwig's Hospital for the full-time position as ophthalmologic surgeon that had just become available. The large hospital was situated in the neighbourhood of the Sophien church, north of Ziegelstrasse. Although Api had worked there occasionally before the war, he doubted that he was going to take up this kind offer. The job would grant him security, but it would also mean that he would have to give up his own practice, which he was loath to do. As Api debated these possibilities, he thought that at least they promised some sense of a future.

One powerful motivation for leaving Berlin Mitte was that life in the Russian zone was becoming increasingly dangerous for a *Pg*. The Soviet occupation was vigorous in its hunt for former members of the Nazi Party. A historian of the period wrote recently: 'The Russians were firm believers in collective guilt and any German was liable for punishment, even death.' The very next day Api heard that a friend, also a member of the Party, had his apartment searched at ten at night and that the little he had left was taken away: jewellery, furniture, a typewriter, even an iron. Living in similar insecurity, Api listened to every step in the house wondering each time whether they came for him. He could not be sure of any neighbour because there were so many denunciations and false accusations among the Berlin population. He was actually more irritated and disgusted by the behaviour of the Germans against each other than by the measures, however strict or senseless, taken by the Russians. 'The German people behave in such a manner among themselves that Russian commandants already have imprisoned denunciators with open expressions of scorn for such a spirit between them.'

Nevertheless, Api felt unable to follow either Dr Hüdepohl's or Frau Grossmann's advice and make a move at that moment. Perhaps his physical condition further undermined his ability to reach a decision. Even though his stomach was improving, he was developing other complaints that troubled him increasingly. He assumed that many of them had to do with malnutrition, such as his bladder pains, cramps from varicose veins in his left leg, hunger edemas on both legs and a bleeding sore in his nose that would not heal. He so feared getting sick before the longed-for reunion.

33

Paradise Lost

One has to be prepared for anything.

O
n Saturday 23 June Api forced himself to make one more of his petitioner's visits in search of eye patients. If he could get enough patients, he might be able to stay in Luisenstrasse after all, which in the end was what was closest to his heart. This time he decided to see Dr Blumann who lived in Dahlem, a place of hundreds of dear memories where Nyussi and he had started out in 1920 as newlyweds. Before he could leave for Dahlem, however, he first had to attend another meeting of doctors at the Health Bureau. After it was over, he took out his borrowed bike and rode off westward.

Along Kurfürstendamm, Api still noticed the ruins of stores and the burnt-out buildings he was used to seeing on the east side of the Tiergarten, but as he turned south things got better. On Hildegardstrasse in Wilmersdorf he noticed only one collapsed house; all the others were intact, ivy grown, with cheerful curtains in the windows. And when he reached Dahlem, he found entire neighbourhoods almost unharmed. The handsome villas shaded by large old beech and linden trees looked as in peacetime. The atmosphere was so different from what he had become used to in Berlin Mitte that he could not believe he was still in the same city. Instead of groups of occupying troops and columns of ragged refugees, here civilians were relaxing in gardens and arbours. It seemed like paradise compared to the grey wilderness he called home.

Seeing this made him wonder anew whether it would not be better to move from the ravaged centre of Berlin. But counter-arguments immediately crowded his mind. First of all, he doubted that it would be possible. Even if it were, he preferred to stay in an area where he was known. Most importantly, he felt such loyalty to the place which had allowed him to climb out of poverty and, with hard work and parsimony, establish a comfortable life for us all. He felt that he already had sacrificed so much and invested all his money to stay and rebuild the Luisenstrasse practice that he could not and would not relinquish it now. For, if he gave up voluntarily, he would have nothing at all. With vigour from that momentary resolution, he pedalled even harder to get to his destination.

Api found Dr Blumann's house undamaged and elegantly furnished. It felt strange to see such unharmed comfort. Dr Blumann was kind and friendly and Api could talk openly to him about his fears and his need of eye patients. At one point Api was moved to say that given his current unimaginably horrible circumstances he was almost happy that Dieter, his son, was not there to live through this. Dr Blumann exclaimed, 'No, no! I cannot imagine if I had to give mine up. Knowing what I would have given for the life of my boy, I can judge your sorrow.' Despite all the sympathy and understanding, Api was glad when the begging visit was over. He was not sure what, if anything, it would bring.

After he left Dr Blumann, Api needed some company. Except for his professional associations he had been alone for too long. On the spur of the moment he decided to visit some old friends, Fritz and Mizzi Hones, who lived nearby at the edge of the Grunewald. He had not seen the couple for many months, perhaps even longer. I vaguely remember those names from Api's stories but I really know nothing about them, except, judging by their location, that they must have been well-to-do. Leaning his bike against a tree of their garden, he knocked at their door. It was a reunion with heartfelt joy on both sides. The Hones lived in a wonderfully green district of suburban villas and gardens bursting with colour. The roses were blooming profusely and spreading their scent to the deck chairs, where the three of them sat around a white table in the middle of a green lawn. The living room had a shiny piano in a cosy corner. Touching a few chords, Api noted that it was playing in tune, not like the piano that he occasionally heard in his attic. How good it felt to be among friends in such beautiful surroundings. Mizzi cooked a tasty dinner in his honour. He wondered where she got all the ingredients, especially the fresh meat and fruit. Fritz fetched a bottle of wine from the cellar to celebrate. They talked much of the past and of us. For Api, who always dreaded his now empty Saturdays, this one, seated among old friends in a green garden, was like paradise; a wonderfully soothing respite. It was also tiring. He had cycled more than 20 miles, thinking with every stroke of the pedal that, if he was cycling to Suderburg, he already would have done almost one-seventh of that journey.

On Sunday Api did not have to go out right away. It was a balmy morning and he spent the early part of it taking an air bath by his attic window, talking with the swallows, the small clouds, with past and future, with us and with his merciful God. Inevitably, his thoughts turned back to the past. He estimated that Nyussi and he had lived through about 1,300 happy and harmonious Sundays, but he worried that there were to be no more.

In better times he would have started every morning with push-ups and stretches. Api was a follower of Dr Kneipp's methods, which the doctor had publicised originally in 1896. Dr Kneipp believed in naturopathy, using nature to help heal the body. His method was synergistic, based on good blood circulation and a toughening of the body. Some of the things Dr Kneipp advocated to fight disease were dipping into icy water or running barefoot through the snow. When I was with Api in the early 1950s, we never went swimming in the winter but he told me that when he was young he used to break the ice and take a dip. After the first snowfall he did, however, urge me to make a quick run with him barefoot across the lawn. Although I resisted at first, it turned out to be an exhilarating experience. We both laughed a lot as we caught our breath with the sudden cold. After a short run we came back inside and, still laughing, dried our pleasantly burning feet.

In these immediate post-war days, Api had neither the strength nor the alacrity of spirit for even the most modest form of exercise. Yet he felt stimulated by his social experience of the day before. He thought of his closest friends, the Sieverts, and decided to make use of his borrowed bike to visit them.

I assume that they had been friends since the 1920s for in an address directory for 1925 both Api and the Sieverts were listed as living at Luisenstrasse 41. I know that later the Sieverts moved into a house of their own. Herr Sievert had been a director at Siemens, the famous electrical company that had a huge industrial complex called Siemens City in the north-west of Berlin. The association with Siemens certainly makes me wonder about Herr Sievert's role under the Nazis, but as far as I remember nothing was ever said about this. I never met him for he died soon after the war, yet I still vividly remember his wife Gerdi, a tiny woman with piercing black eyes. Seeing her, I was always surprised how her large nose dominated her face and how her smile transformed her sharp features. Even when I knew her as an elderly woman she was spirited and full of life. Before she came to visit us in the 1950s, my grandmother told me that Gerdi had been an adventurer when she was young. She was one of the first women to study at the university in Königsberg, the home town of Immanuel Kant. After graduation in 1914, she went on a tour of Siberia all by herself and she was there when the First World War broke out. Gerdi made her way back to Prussia through enemy land and seemed to have relished the danger and the adventure. In Berlin, the Sieverts, who were childless, spoiled my mother and uncle and served as a surrogate family. When Gerdi died in the 1970s she willed what she had left in valuables, a few pieces of jewellery and a silk oriental rug, to my mother.

The two old friends were glad to see Api and did what they could to cheer him up. They even set a picture of Api and Nyussi on the coffee table. It was taken on holiday in the Riesengebirge, a mountain range between Silesia and Bohemia, which was a favourite destination for Berliners. My grandparents had always liked rugged mountain hikes and Api remembered that this one in late autumn had been particularly challenging. I also have a picture from that trip, and like to think that it is the same one Api looked at so fondly. Nyussi looks dashing in a long black coat with little black ankle boots and a jaunty hat, and Api is wearing once again his favourite knickerbockers and a jacket. It did Api good to see his wife in happier times and it hurt him at the same time. Seeing his pale and thin face, and remembering his sweet tooth, the Sieverts made sure to feed Api some cake and bread with jam. After an ample coffee hour, they had liqueurs and even champagne.

Delighting in the company of friends and the conversation of old times, Api stayed from 3.30 p.m. until 8.30 p.m. He had always derived an almost childlike pleasure from parties and social gatherings of all sorts and used to be a great one for entertaining his visitors with funny stories. Now he rarely even smiled. Even here, surrounded by the warmth of old friendship, the ominous present never left him entirely. When it came time to say goodbye, he gave his friendly hosts our address, 'just in case' – implying that he might not survive to see us again. He added apologetically: 'One has to be prepared for anything.'

Api cycled home accompanied by the fragrance of the linden trees. It had been Nyussi's favourite time. Upon reaching his attic, his first glance was out the window at the sky. 'The evening sky – still without moon, but of a depth and softness which could even put a less longing person into a sentimental mood, a few thunder clouds, silent and immovable and my evening swallows.' It had been a good day, although he had cycled another 20 miles. As he remembered the pleasant evening and thought of Nyussi's picture on the Sieverts' table, Api noted down the details of his visit, ending with, 'We even had some *Pezsgö*', which means bubbly in Hungarian. With one more glance in our direction to the north-west, he bade us goodnight. That evening he dropped off to sleep right away without the aid of any pills.

Thinking back over his weekend the following morning, Api appreciated how lucky he was. He was treated to the occasional good meal, and he still had some friends who helped him out. He thought about the tired people he had seen trudging to work across the Tiergarten, who had nothing to eat at the end of it. Several areas had not received a single gram of fat for four to six weeks. Api understood that it was not easy to provision a destroyed city of, still, 2.5 million people, but he also felt that it should not be such an insurmountable problem for the Russians. Yet with the passing days the food supply seemed to him to get worse, not better.

The days and weeks of the summer passed without bringing Api closer to a decision. On 25 June he reflected in his diary that 'tomorrow, Tuesday, it will be eleven terrible desolate weeks since our most awful good bye in Suderburg'. He had been right when he had been certain that the war could not last more than four weeks. But how wrong, how naïvely wrong he had been in imagining that, should we have survived the catastrophe, we would be reunited immediately. There still was no sign that the postal blockade would end and Api was afraid of the approaching winter. The 21 June, the longest day of the year, had already passed. It had been a summer of rare beauty, and yet how unimaginably horrible it had been, but, he admonished us as he wrote, 'don't let your sorrow stop you from praying'. Without prayer he himself could not go on.

34

The Little Swallows Play

Everything breathes God's peace and infinity, and
makes the sorrows of this world, where so many, so
infinitely many people give up and despair, appear
small and trivial.

Every day throughout June the newspapers continued their
denunciations of fellow Germans: 'The newspaper falls all over
itself in its smear campaign against *Pgs* and creates a dangerous
atmosphere for everyone, whether active, inactive, or opposed!' As a
Pg, Api had to fill out a lengthy application and then submit to questioning at
the employment office in order to be able to work as a doctor. He felt mortified
by the process, but knew that he had to do it. The one reassuring news item
in June was that in the British and American occupation zones of Germany
the situation was not nearly as bad as in Berlin under the Russians. He hoped,
therefore, that we in Suderburg were faring better than he was in Berlin. Api
would have liked to talk to us about the situation, but did not think it was
possible to discuss politics in his letters. All he wrote in his diary was that he
was convinced that 'peace and prosperity are unthinkable without a return
to piety, of Christian brotherly love, mutual tolerance, in short, human ethics,
in our enemies and in our own people. And that,' he added, 'still looks pretty
bad, especially with our own people.'

At the end of June the weather was turning chilly and windy. It reminded Api of the mountain hikes he and Nyussi had taken in the Riesengebirge, but it also heightened his fears of the cold to come. The morning of Friday 29 June brought two unwelcome discoveries. When he went to his favourite spot, a lookout toward the north-west in the direction of Suderburg on the first floor of the North Sanatorium, he found it bricked up. It used to be his first destination every morning from where he sent his greetings our way. He knew that he would miss that imaginary connection to us. Continuing on to the university clinic for the class with Professor Löhlein, Api discovered that his medical texts had all been stolen. He knew that there was no appeal since a *Pg* had no rights. All his beautiful leather-bound books were gone. The only textbook that was left was one he had worked through twice already.

For a good part of the last weekend in June Api hid away in his attic. It gave him a few hours of unmolested time to think backwards, dreaming of happy Saturdays past. Remembering that it was just about two years ago that we had received news of the death of my father, and that my mother's birthday was coming up on 24 July, Api started a long letter to her to which he planned to add in the next days, just as he had done for Nyussi's birthday. After attending church, Api went to the cemetery to visit his mother's grave for the first time in months. She had died in 1944 and he had been used to going to her grave every few weeks. It was a particularly sad bike ride to her grave as he remembered the many trips we all had made there together. Just a year earlier his son had still been with him. He passed the spot where a stranger had come up and helped with one of the suitcases as we were fleeing from Berlin on our way to the train in February 1945. Now the streets were empty and frightening, made unsafe by drunk and marauding Russian soldiers.

Back home on Sunday afternoon, Api watched aircraft fly overhead and heard the whistle of locomotives. Occasionally he even noticed a civilian car drive down the narrow middle of the street between the rubble. So much motion, yet he was imprisoned and could not budge. The prospect of next Monday's meeting at the employment office, where he had to present his application, worried and humiliated him. He now wrote in his diary only at night because when he got up in the morning he was too depressed even for that.

In peacetime Api had not often dreamt at night, or at least had not remembered his dreams, but now he had vivid dreams almost every night, which tore him out of sleep and disquieted him. They all had to do with confused and failed journeys where nothing worked out and where he never reached his destination. These nightmares were made up from contradictory snippets of information he had picked up during the day. He heard that, beginning on 1 July, only a few days hence, the passage across the River Elbe would be free, or that in exchange for cigarettes you could get a ferry to take you across. Then again someone said that the British would send you back after taking everything you had, or that there were camps of 1,000 people and more, all waiting for an opportunity to get on a train.

That evening he sat by the window, took out his green diary and wrote:

Between some rough rain clouds, the evening descends already noticeably earlier over the sad hopelessness of the fields of rubble stretching for kilometres and over bent and askew rafters which are still standing here and there and which grin above it ironically. But the little swallows play, screaming happily as in my childhood, and the small high altitude clouds which pass in front of blue islands in the sky still breathe peace and preach God's merciful father's will.

However, then his mind turned to us and he became afraid:

Sometimes I imagine the worst, the thought that perhaps all my longing, my prayers, my fight against my weakness, against myself, for this my only wish for the future is already meeting emptiness because something has happened to you, my dearest ones!! I am also unhappy that there is no possibility to release you of the same worry about myself.

At this point Api felt that even words and language, which had always helped him deal with difficult and painful as well as happy times, were deserting him:

Oh, if I still had the concentration and the knack for language to describe to you in a poem what longing can make of a poor human

178

soul. Such a string of wonderful days we have not had for many years. The sky is densely sown with 'little sheep' [the term Germans use to describe the fluffy cumulus clouds]. Everything breathes God's peace and infinity, and makes the sorrows of this world, where so many, so infinitely many people give up and despair, appear small and trivial. If only one could flee to it!! But this world of misery forces one to take in, with each step, unimaginably sad, heartrending pictures: amidst the tortured, tired, starved and fearful faces of almost everyone, one sees groups laden with parcels, dressed in tatters, deathly exhausted. They crouch on front stoops, dumb and blind to what goes on around them, almost ashamed of their nameless misery, not daring to raise their eyes above the ground, devoid of any hope because they recognize that even with the best of will no one can help them in any way. And therefore I have, besides my divided desire to have you with me before one knows what will happen, the racing fear that you could also have set out and become part of such a totally despairing situation! Remain strong in your dear love and in your trust in God!

Api felt at one moment that he could do anything if only we were there to work for, but the very next he was overcome with a feeling of abandonment, fearing that he could not go on. He was so afraid that, even in the worst-case scenario, if he was near the end, there would be no possibility to hurry to us for a last goodbye.

35

Without the Faintest Guilt

A people who allow such a thing cannot count on our compassion!

S tarting in June, people had to submit requests for 'de-Nazification' in order to be able to return to their previous positions. Such requests, made to a special committee of the magistrate, had to include testimonies by colleagues, neighbours or family members. The result, if successful, was popularly known as the *Persilschein*, the Persil certificate. Persil was the brand name of a well-known washing powder, which boasted that it would make everything spotless.

Api had no *Persilschein* and at this point did not seem to have tried for one. As a *Pg* he felt persecuted. He lived in fear and saw no way of re-establishing himself. The constant insecurity wore him down and yet, he reflected, 'And all that without the faintest guilt, but on the other hand again that is a great consolation and support'. This sentence appears in his diary without preparation or further comment, but it is linked to other statements scattered throughout which stress that he never did harm to anyone and that he never succeeded because of another's misfortune.

Reading this, I am confronted again with my key quandary, this time expressed as unambiguously as never before, 'without the faintest guilt'. Api did not feel guilty or in any way implicated in the murder and destruction perpetrated by the Nazi regime. I realise that he was not personally responsible for any of it and that, apart from having joined the Party on 1 May 1933, he did nothing further to advance its cause; he did not hold any office in the Party or persecute anyone. Nevertheless, he had been a member of the Party and had been there and witnessed persecution: noticed the 'No Jews Allowed' signs on park benches and cinemas, seen his Jewish colleagues disappear. I am not imagining that I would have been able to do anything more than Api did, for I know myself not to be brave. I also have no idea how far his resistance did or didn't go at the time, what little acts of courage he was able to perform. I cannot sit in judgement over a man I knew to be compassionate and tolerant. For the moment – and I know that this subject will not let me go – I feel that if there was guilt it would have to be such as each individual has to work out with his or her own conscience. I understand why this was not the time for Api to engage in such additional torture, but instead seek any consolation he could find.

The immediate post-war world did not allow Api to hide from this issue of German guilt, however. A problem that nagged Api constantly was whether he should make a request for what he called the political *Unbedenklichkeitserklärung*, literally a 'declaration of no objection'. I am not sure whether Api was referring to the de-Nazification document, the *Persilschein*, or whether there was some earlier clearance form that Party members had to fill out before they could get permission to move from one occupation zone to another, or leave Berlin altogether. Api had no idea whether it would help him if he applied for this document or whether, on the contrary, it would damage his prospects or draw unnecessary attention to himself. He thought about this back and forth as soon as he woke up in the morning, and had to pull himself together to break this pointless spiral and get up at all. Thinking of Nyussi, he said to himself, 'I was so spoiled by you and our beloved togetherness where we talked about and decided everything together.'

About the same time, Professor Seegert, whom Api often assisted in operations, told him that a British major was reported to have said after his visit to a concentration camp: 'A people who allow such a thing cannot count on our compassion!' Api commented in despair: 'As if they didn't know that any rebellious word had meant death, without helping in the slightest.'

To me today, both Api's and the major's reactions are understandable. Api probably did not know about the concentration camps before May 1945 and he had tried to live his life helping, not hurting, others. At the same time, the major who had just witnessed the horror of such a camp must have been overwhelmed by that experience and thought of the perpetrators as inhuman. A booklet handed out to British and Commonwealth troops adopted the same hostile attitude to the Germans. It said, 'the Germans have only themselves to blame'. Similarly, the *Stars and Stripes* admonished its soldiers: 'Don't get chummy with Jerry. In heart, body and spirit, every German is a Hitler.' The Allies, especially the British and Americans, wanted to make sure that there was no fraternisation between their troops and the German population and that Allied soldiers did not take pity on the people's suffering. One reason given for the interdiction to fraternise was the continued Allied fear of Operation Werwolf. Historian David Stafford, however, suggests that 'the main purpose of the ban was to make it clear to the Germans that they were a nation guilty of aggression and criminality and had made themselves pariahs and outcasts of the civilized world.'

36

The Allies are Coming

Everyone waits and expects something from the
Anglo-Americans. Not me. There is only one thing
I long for right now with all my heart: postal service.

At the beginning of July 50,000 soldiers from the US
82nd Airborne Division and the British 7th Armoured Division
reached Berlin and afterwards the city was divided into four
occupation zones. The eastern part of Berlin from Mitte to
Treptow stayed in Russian hands. On the western side – all of which later
would be called West Berlin – were the French, British and American zones.
The French occupied Wedding and Reinickendorf in the north; the British
were below that in Tiergarten, Charlottenburg and Wilmersdorf; and the
Americans had the south-western part of Berlin including Tempelhof and
Steglitz.

For people caught in the Russian sector, however, little changed after this
new arrangement. In fact, for Api things got worse. The hunt for *Pgs*, Party
members, only heated up in July. It made Api live in constant fear of arrest
and deportation, and in time it would leave him homeless. NSDAP members
continued to be fired from public offices. The Berlin magistrate resolved to
dismiss all doctors who had been members of any of Hitler's special forces –
the SS, Gestapo or SA – or who had shown themselves otherwise 'unworthy'.

Pg doctors who were still allowed to work could do so only conditionally and for limited times. They were to be paid 0.72 Reichsmarks an hour, the same as workers in the rubble fields.

Api worried ever more seriously about his *Pg* status. He never mentioned the pay but he was concerned about food. He had received the lowest ration card. Cards were distributed according to five classes of people: heavy labourers, public officials, doctors, pastors, industrialists and artists were to be at the top in Group 1; Group 2 were blue-collar workers; Group 3 were white-collar workers; Group 4 included children up to 15 years; and in Group 5, 'Others', were *Pgs* and the unemployed. Group 5, by the way, also included housewives. The day's rations for Api consisted of 7g fat, 20g meat, 300g bread, 30g grain, 15g sugar and 400g potatoes – but even that was guaranteed only on paper and, the fat especially, rarely materialised.

On Monday morning, 2 July, Api got up early and went out before breakfast to try to assess what the new resolutions against *Pgs* meant for him. First he went to see if he could not move up in his ration card classification. After a two-hour wait he succeeded and was moved up to Group 1, an indication that he was not on any 'unworthy' list. This meant a little more of everything, especially fat, if available. Api's next errand was to report to the Health Bureau. When he wrote about it later in his diary, he entered only the words 'paragraph 218'. He obviously did not want to talk about this issue, even in the intimacy of his diary, just as he had not mentioned rape. Paragraph 218 referred to the law that forbade doctors to perform abortions. Doctors in Berlin, however, quickly decided to suspend paragraph 218 temporarily and perform abortions on the great number of raped women who had unwanted pregnancies. This virtual suspension of paragraph 218 soon was extended to many Western zones. In this doctors had the support of the Protestant but not of the Catholic Church. Some critics, however, have seen this measure simply as 'a continuation of Nazi-sanctioned abortions in case of rape by foreigners in order to preserve the purity of the race'.

After the Health Bureau, Api could not put off his next errand any longer. He had to appear at the employment office to register in person, as was required, and hand in his application to work in his profession. Despite having spent the weekend anxious about this, permission was granted right away. The need for doctors in Berlin, coupled with his status as an inactive Party member, allowed him to continue to work as a doctor. But he could not be sure whether that would remain so in the future. As he had been told at the Health Bureau, there were no assurances for the safety of his equipment should he open his own practice. 'Anyone,' the official had told him, 'can take anything away from a *Pg*.'

Api had also read about a new decree to confiscate the possessions of *Pgs* from former block captains up. The Nazis had organised the entire city down to each street, to which block captains had been assigned. Although Api had never even been a block captain, he was sorry for those among them who had done no harm to anyone and yet had to suffer this hardship. What annoyed Api particularly was that all these decrees and resolutions failed to take into account the many non-*Pgs* who had been active during the Nazi regime. Without being members of the Party, they had hurt and betrayed innocent people. The actual situation under Hitler, as in any totalitarian regime, was much more complex and ambiguous than these new regulations seemed to allow. But at least for the moment the dreaded meeting at the employment office was over. It had gone more smoothly and quickly than Api had hoped, and he left the office with the desired work approval, relieved that the whole thing was behind him.

Next, Api had to go to the Office of Work Deployment in order to obtain his release from shovelling rubble for the month of July, another chore imposed on *Pgs*. It, too, was granted right away. So all together, and despite all the nervous energy and the time spent running around and waiting in offices, it had not been too bad a day.

Waiting in offices, Api noticed a new mood of expectancy. People had high hopes that conditions would change now that the Americans were in town. He wrote that night:

Everyone waits and expects something from the Anglo-Americans. Not me. There is only one thing I long for with all my heart: postal service ... How many times every day my heart constricts in sudden pain when the locomotives whistle, cars or airplanes roar toward the west, and the immediate thought 'imprisoned' grinds into nothing every dream of a reunion and all the heartrending stormy tender wishes.

The summer was passing and the span of life God still allowed him seemed to melt away in loneliness. The shorter days also made him think anxiously about the coming winter. The stored coal had all been devoured by fire during the bombing raids, and without coal and food it would get even worse in Berlin and cost many more lives.

There was one bit of good news going around. It was said that, as of now, Berliners could send greetings to faraway family via radio. Api resolved to cycle to the radio station the very next day. On Saturday, he showed up at the station as soon as they opened in the morning. He entered his name for the programme *Your relatives in the Reich send greetings* ... but since he doubted that we had a radio to hear this message he also wrote a postcard. He had heard that postcards in English or German would get forwarded by the occupation if they were written in the modern Latin and not in the old German *Sütterlin* script. Api did not use the old script, yet even in the late 1940s I was taught the *Sütterlin* script in school. When we finally got to use the more fluid and rounded Latin script in school, I saw it as a sign of having grown up. However, we were still using a nib pen and I remember the teacher telling us over and over 'thin up, heavy down', meaning a light stroke for the letters that went above the line and a strong one for those that reached below it. Although we had to practise this again and again, I never mastered the art. My knowledge of the old German script did come in handy, however, when I was deciphering the letters of nineteenth-century immigrants for books I was writing about that period. The generation after me, however, cannot write or read it any better than could the Allies back then.

Rumour, which still was the main currency, had it that the entire Luisenstrasse was to be taken over by the Russians for their military offices. The government buildings on Wilhelmstrasse were in ruins and would not have been used anyway since they represented Nazi rule. So the Russians settled on the nearby Luisenstrasse for their central command. It, too, had many large official buildings, even though they needed repair. Already the Russians had taken over both the Langenbeck-Virchow House at Luisenstrasse 58, just a block from Api's practice, and the nearby Leitz and Zeiss Building for the headquarters of the *GPU*, the much-feared Soviet secret police. The veterinary college next to the Langenbeck-Virchow House served as Russian command headquarters. Other buildings on Luisenstrasse had also been taken over, so that Api was surrounded by the Soviet administration.

If more was to come and the whole street was to be closed to locals, Api would have to act quickly to take everything out of his surgery. But where, he wondered, could he go with the little he had left? Where in this devastated city could he possibly find a place? He saw so many who wandered about the streets without shelter, without home. He wondered, 'to where on earth could I find safekeeping for the last concrete remains and mementos of our sunny past?' By Frau Grossmann's accounts things were better in Steglitz or Friedenau in the American occupation zone, and he had seen for himself how intact the streets of Dahlem were, now in the British sector. If only he did not have to live in the Russian zone!

'Oh, my best ones, if at least I could have your advice in this desperate situation, encouragement and your love around me. You cannot imagine my dilemma and my besieged desolation.' Api wrote this, sitting by the open window of his surgery and waiting fruitlessly for at least one patient to show up. Just then 'in a screaming irony, a jazz band drones on in a cheap bar which just has opened nearby and people dance on the volcano either thoughtlessly or with gallows humour'. Api felt once more that he was living by day the nightmares of his chaotic travel dreams. Next the sky turned black and a thunderstorm drenched his waiting room and surgery and turned both into a lake. Api was totally discouraged. All his work had been for naught. Help was impossible to get since all the masons and carpenters of the area were employed by the Russians. When he got back to his attic room, it too had been flooded. The five pails and washbowls he had set out could not handle the torrents of water.

The futility of everything, his continued ill health and constant hunger paired with his personal insecurity, wore him down so that he could hardly drag himself about. At this stage Api was so afraid that something would happen to him before he could see us again that he went downstairs to the North Sanatorium and entrusted his diary to the head nurse for safe keeping. Under no circumstances did he want it to get lost to us. 'For,' he wrote quickly before handing the diary over, 'even if much of it is very repetitive, some of it is quite interesting.' However, he retrieved his green diary just a couple of days later for he needed to continue his daily reports and conversation with us.

Api had borrowed some medical texts from the Ziegelstrasse clinic and had intended to study them over the weekend. Some were in French and he was pleased that he could read them still as fluently as the German ones. But under the new and frightening prospect of becoming homeless, he decided to abandon his books for the weekend and use the time to cycle around from acquaintance to acquaintance, begging for help in finding asylum. He did not have much hope of success since the few people he still knew who had survived also had nothing to help him with. His pride suffered again with this begging errand but he saw no other choice. To help him fall asleep and gain some strength for the next day he dosed himself heavily with sleeping pills.

The weekend excursions were as fruitless as he had feared. On his journeys Api noticed the first American tanks in the streets of Berlin Mitte. He could only admire the wonderful newness of these machines from their antennas down to their treads. They looked as if they had just rolled off the factory floor. He marvelled again how Hitler and his group could have imagined standing up against such overwhelming force with their make-do weapons and unarmed *Volkssturm* troops of boys and old men.

Tuesday 10 July, Api thought yet again of another anniversary of our parting, now ninety-one days, or thirteen weeks, ago. Unable to do any major repairs or improvements to his attic, he bought two red impatiens plants for his window. As he set them down on the sill he reflected how much had changed in his life, and yet how nature continued on its accustomed course:

> The sky is the same as before, in meadows and fields there is the same blossoming and will to life, the swallows whirr, the butterflies dance, and the coloured flies stand above fragrant blossoms, just as in my childhood. And the souls of men are just as they were 1000 years ago, full of hopes and desires, of worries and prayers. And yet now they are so totally broken! People beg in the streets for a piece of dry bread.

Gazing out of his attic window lost in such thoughts, Api's attention was drawn to a woman across the street. She sat by her window, chewing a piece of dry bread. Then he noticed someone coming into the room behind her and Api watched as the woman quickly leaned down to hide the piece of bread on the sill below her. As he wrote about what he had just witnessed, he ended with two exclamation points to suggest the shock he felt about such mean behaviour.

37

Another Dismissal

You have your own practice now and no longer need
this work.

On Wednesday 11 July, Api suffered another blow similar to his altercation with Dr Kleberger. Professor Löhlein dismissed him. He explained his action by saying, 'after all, you have your own practice now and no longer need this work'. But then he added something that greatly perturbed Api, although he did not understand its implication. As he tried to record what Professor Löhlein had said, he could not even remember the exact words, so great had been his agitation. Professor Löhlein had mentioned something about a warlike atmosphere and whether Api had also noticed this. It is not clear to me, and Api himself did not understand what Professor Löhlein meant, except that it seemed to him a veiled accusation of something Api had said or done that had caused tension and this 'warlike atmosphere'. The very phrase was loaded, especially in July 1945, barely ten weeks after the end of the Second World War. Professor Löhlein concluded the interview by repeating, 'Well, to make it short, you have after all your own practice now ...'

For days afterwards Api wracked his brain but could not think of anything he had said or done to offend the professor or anyone around him. He was prostrate. Two months ago, he thought, he was still physically and mentally in better shape to withstand such a shock. Now he was not so sure. He felt cowardly and fainthearted. The dismissal made him feel more helpless and insecure, afraid even to leave his own four walls and shy of meeting people and of doing or saying anything at all. He trembled to get up each morning because it was the beginning of a day which would come to him with all kinds of decisions – and mistakes – to be made.

Although shaken and fundamentally unsure of himself, Api resolved not to give in or give up. After all, he still had occasional work assisting Professor Seegert in operations at the women's clinic of the Ziegelstrasse complex, and he also continued to work at the North Sanatorium despite the row with Dr Kleberger. In fact he was already scheduled to assist in an operation there to remove an intestinal obstruction. Api also admonished himself to heed the lessons of his youth, which he had instilled in his own children. He needed to continue to work intensively and further his education. So to regain his mental balance, Api turned to his borrowed eye surgery texts. He ended the day with a little more hope thinking that again one day, a bad one, was past and perhaps it had brought him one day closer to a reunion with us.

Nevertheless, the next morning Api continued to brood on the dismissal. It had been so unexpected and he wondered why it had happened and whether he had been responsible in any way. He had tried so very hard not to offend anyone and always anxiously weighed his actions and words. He just could not think of anything he had said or done. The situation further undermined his self-confidence, so much so that on Friday 13 July Api was scared because of the date alone. He was ashamed of this. He felt that it was a sign of how frightened and cowardly he had become, and he would not tell this to anyone except us in his diary. As if to confirm his fear, the morning brought a downpour that set his attic room afloat yet again – only the impatiens on the windowsill were glad for the water. To add to the ominous mood, he heard a little child cry with an ever weaker voice from a building across the street. Api feared that the child would not live much longer. On that inauspicious Friday the 13th, Api also had to take care of a patient who was suspected of having typhoid. Although he regularly treated such patients, that day he worried about contagion. Proper sanitation was not yet available and thousands of nasty big dung flies continued to plague the city. People devoted hours to killing as many as they could, but their numbers continued to grow.

As I kept reading about the plague of flies, I had to think of Sartre's recasting of the Orestes tragedy in *The Flies*. Although the play was written two years earlier in 1943, perhaps flies had plagued Paris then as well. Or it was an eerily prophetic play with its characters haunted by the fateful flies.

At this low point Professor Seegert came to the rescue. He presented him with a ticket for the following day's 5.30 p.m. performance of Schiller's *The Parasite* at the Deutsches Theatre. He knew how much Api had enjoyed the theatre and was trying to cheer him up. The Deutsches Theatre had been reopened as a theatre on 26 June with a performance of *Nathan the Wise*. Lessing's classic had been forbidden under the Nazis and now its language of humanity and tolerance spoke directly, if painfully, to the audience.

I had never heard of Schiller's *The Parasite*, but thanks to the wonders of the internet I found it pretty quickly. It is a five-act comedy called *The Parasite or the Art to Make One's Fortune*. I never thought of Schiller as a writer of comedies, and this one probably is best forgotten. The play is set in eighteenth-century Paris and has just one set: Minister Narbonne's antechamber in which the comedy of love and intrigue unfolds. It is a light play, yet I imagine that some of its statements may have reverberated with the audience, such as talk about 'the abuses of the late government' and its final line that 'justice exists only on stage'. Api may have felt close to one bit of poetry, albeit bad, which reflected his own state of mind. The 17-year-old heroine recites these lines:

> *But these thousand voices*
> *Of the awakening nature*
> *Awaken in the depth of my bosom*
> *Only the heaviest grief!*

The Sunday after the Schiller performance, Api felt a recurrence of his stomach ailment. He had never recovered completely but now it grew worse again. He decided that although he was weak, he would not miss church. The short walk to the Sophien church exhausted him, however, so much so that he almost collapsed during the service. He had to lower his head on to the pew in front of him until the spell passed. For once he did not remember much of the sermon. Nevertheless, after the service he got on his bike as planned and rode off in the direction of Tempelhof and Friedenau to see Frau Grossmann. The fresh air, he thought, would only do him good. Unfortunately he had a different bike, the previous one having been returned to its owner, and this one was much harder to peddle and the tyres lost air several times on the way. When he reached his destination pretty worn out, he was rewarded with an excellent lunch of sour braten and gooseberry compote, followed by coffee and cake. Although the cake was baked without fat or sugar and the coffee was *Muckefuck*, they were both treats to be enjoyed as a rarity.

The days of the summer passed in the same deadening routine. The heat was becoming oppressive again, which increased the threat of epidemics. Then Api found his son's birth certificate, which brought on another bout of pain and uncertainties. Should he leave? Wouldn't his dear son's advice to him be 'to just take off'? A thousand reasons urged him to grab his always ready rucksack and start hiking, but invariably there were other equally emotional reasons that made him stay. He was so very attached to the place where he had built his life, and he also did not want to give the impression that he was running away.

Then again, summer was passing and the general situation, instead of getting calmer, deteriorated into always new and more serious aggravations. Also, his physical condition worsened almost every day and he soon would be too weak to set out at all, if he was not so already. His isolation terrified him and he felt unable to make such a life-altering decision all alone.

38

Homeless

*No need to write down everything that is going on with
me and within me, I will not ever forget it anyhow.*

The middle of July brought dramatic changes for Germany, and for Api personally. It was the time of the Potsdam Conference. Api remembered that it was also in Potsdam where the inauguration of Hitler as chancellor had taken place twelve years ago, when he had cherished such hopes for a new beginning. Perhaps this time it would come true. Api was concerned about reports that Stalin would not participate and that the conference had been cancelled. He saw the Potsdam Conference as one ray of hope for the future. Along with most Germans, Api was glad when he heard that Churchill and Truman had arrived in Berlin on Monday 16 July. The meeting started the following day at Cecilienhof, the former home of Crown Prince Wilhelm Hohenzollern. Stalin, Truman and Churchill met for two weeks to work out the fate of Germany and decide the future of Europe.

The night Churchill and Truman arrived in Berlin, the Sieverts happened to throw a birthday party. Api took the rickety bike again and made his laborious way to them dressed in his best clothes, the striped trousers and black jacket, which he had carefully brushed after the last bike trip. Even so, the black jacket was looking less black than it had when Herr Gerhardt had given it to him. He added his pearl tiepin as a final touch. He felt frail and shaky, but he would not miss the party. He also looked forward to the food, for with all the days of feeling sick to his stomach, he had not realised that he was hungry. The Sieverts also offered cigars, cognac and champagne, all of which they somehow had rescued from before the war. Api enjoyed the moment of luxury and cordially thanked his hosts.

Amidst all his misery, he often expressed a deep gratitude for what he had and what others did for him; a pervasive sense of gratitude which he also instilled in me. Api never forgot those who were hungry and had nothing, which he knew was the condition of the majority of people around him. It made him feel guilty that he was allowed to enjoy such a feast. Yet neither here nor elsewhere did he attribute his good fortune to the always powerful advantages of class standing. As Api cycled back, still warmed by good food and cognac, and with a strong wind from the east pushing him along, he imagined that he could be in Suderburg in fifteen hours. More realistically, he planned to follow the Sieverts' suggestion and consult a Frau Paterek at the Housing Bureau on Breitenbachplatz about a place to stay in the American zone.

Action was forced on him sooner than he had anticipated. On Thursday 19 July, Api had to give up his last asylum, his little 'swallow's nest', because water was coming in everywhere. All the containers he had used to keep it at bay proved useless against the ever-increasing number of leaks. There was no hope, either, of getting patients to come to Luisenstrasse since it was dominated by the Russian military. Hardly any civilians were left there. Building by building, the entire street was being requisitioned by the Soviets for army quarters. People who used to live on the street had either escaped with whatever they could carry or were thrown out. Last, but by no means least, was Api's fear of arrest. Word or rumour had come to him that the Soviet secret police, whose headquarters were just a few feet away on Luisenstrasse, had inquired about him. Api did not know why or what it was about or even if it was true, but the suggestion alone was enough to scare him.

Api had good reason to be afraid. The Soviet secret police, or *GPU*, arrested thousands of civilians in Berlin after the war. People were interrogated in the notorious *GPU* cellars, where they were subjected to threats and torture in an effort to extract incriminating statements. As a doctor Api might not end up in a labour camp, but arrest and transportation to somewhere in the East was hardly a less-frightening prospect. For weeks he had listened anxiously to every knock on his door; he never went to sleep without the thought that they may come for him that night and he had his clothes always ready for immediate departure.

Therefore, on 19 July, with a heavy heart and great foreboding, Api scribbled in his diary: 'No need to write down everything that is going on with me and within me, I will not ever forget it anyhow. Is what I am doing wise or unwise? This time I am doing what others advise me rather unanimously.' Api shouldered his rucksack and went in search of a place to stay. He had picked out his most important instruments, especially the little mirrors with which he examined his patients' eyes, along with some books, a shirt, a tie, his best jacket and trousers, some underwear and, of course, his tiepin. Out on the streets he felt truly homeless, just like the streams of pitiful refugees for whom he had been so sorry. Api almost had to laugh at what a fool he had been to imagine that he could create even a small livelihood out of the rubble in the middle of Berlin.

Cut off from the provisions of the clinic and the charity of the nurses there, Api had to forage for food on his own. It was a new experience. He went from one restaurant to another, but most of them were still closed. The few that were open had nothing to offer. At best they served coffee and soda water. Dragging his heavy load, he called upon colleagues and acquaintances. At half past ten that night he stopped at the district housing office, in vain. After that he begged a bed for the night from a friend.

The next morning Api went to see Frau Paterek on Breitenbachplatz, the person the Sieverts had mentioned. It was only a few days ago, but now it seemed an age. On his way there he saw an old woman collapse. She was just another in the heartrending columns of misery; refugees with no place to go. He realised then that although he too had no home, he still was undeservedly fortunate compared with such anguish. Breitenbachplatz, 6km (about 4 miles) south of Berlin Mitte, was in comparatively good shape. Seeing building after building still standing unharmed, he felt 'a moment of envious comparison: if one had lived in such an area, perhaps one could have saved one's stuff which one had grown so fond of!'

Frau Paterek offered him a room in her apartment on Opitzstrasse 3 in Steglitz, not far from Breitenbachplatz. She said that he could move there the next day but made it clear that it was only a temporary arrangement. She wanted to help him out because the Sieverts had told her how much he needed assistance at this moment. Api was relieved that he had a place to stay and leave his luggage at least for a few nights. In the evening he went back to the friendly Dr Blumann whose advice, Api wrote, was 'not in writing!' I do not know what that refers to, whether Dr Blumann was speaking of an application for de-Nazification or a request to move out of the Russian sector, or whether Api had asked Dr Blumann to make some kind of statement on his behalf.

From here on in his diary Api was becoming ever more distraught, almost incapable of forming coherent thoughts and plans. Even his handwriting, always so neat and precise, disintegrated and became shaky and disjointed. He often scratched out words and lines in his diary. He who had always relied on banishing anxiety by putting it into words, now often could not write at all.

In this shaken state Api made his way to his new room. Frau Paterek, the landlady, met him with a warm smile. It did him good to receive such a cordial welcome. The room she had for him was tiny but there were trees right in front of the window, real green shady trees as had not surrounded him since Suderburg. In Berlin Mitte there had been only bits of grass and weeds that struggled to poke their heads out of cracks between ruins. He could tell the time when a building had been destroyed by how tall the weeds had grown. Those that had been ruins for the longest time even had some young saplings emerging from the weeds. Looking out of the window of his room in Steglitz it seemed to Api for the first time that peace had really come. But there were also warning signs of winter cold not far away. The oaks that lined the street were already showing acorns, which meant the beginning of autumn and with it the worry about finding heating materials. Above all else, he feared that the approaching winter made his journey to Suderburg ever more unlikely.

Api unpacked his rucksack. It was not a big task since he had so few belongings left to him. He carefully smoothed out the jacket and trousers Herr Gerhardt had given him and hung them over the one chair in his room. Strangely, at the bottom of his rucksack he had put three children's books, my *Birds of the Woods*, *The Elephant Book* and *Ten Little Negroes*, which he laid on the bedside table next to his one remaining medical text. Just when he wondered what to do next, Frau Paterek knocked on his door and invited him to share her lunch of fried potatoes and tea. He accepted gratefully. Before turning in that night, Api looked at the sky: 'Exquisite light-framed cumulus clouds drift above the wonderful green of the trees and above the silent village peace.' As he lay down in a strange bed, grateful to have a place to put his head, he wondered what he would dream. As superstition has it, whatever you dream the first night in a new place will come true.

Api never recorded any dreams he may have had. In fact, the next day, 21 July, he did not have sufficient concentration to write at all. Before going out in the morning he sat down briefly with his diary but could not find words for his situation. He started to put something down but immediately blacked it all out again. He felt weak and ill and very old. His foot was swollen and he suffered from an inflammation of the veins. He could hardly walk. He thought despairingly that once again he had made the wrong decision by coming to this place. For this one temporary room would not offer any opportunity to start again. He was more uprooted than ever before now that he had given up his last anchor, the place that had been home for so many years.

The following day Api went back one more time to Dr Blumann, who had been so kind before and given him sound advice. They discussed where best to settle. Dr Blumann mentioned the well-to-do districts of Breitenbachplatz and Friedenau, just north of Steglitz. As Api had seen for himself, these areas south of the centre of Berlin had sustained relatively little damage. He knew that they always had been solid middle-class districts where he could hope to start a practice. It felt good to be able to talk to someone about the possibility of a better future. For a brief moment this friendly and personal exchange diverted Api from all the fateful thoughts that haunted him almost to breaking point. Together, they finally settled on Friedenau as the best prospect since Dr Blumann thought he might be able to help Api rent a three-room apartment in that area. Only, he added, one inside wall was missing. So, Api thought, he might have a practice in Friedenau after all, twenty years after he had first considered it.

In the evening Api realised that this had been one of very few Sundays that he had not gone to church and it came at a particularly perilous time for him. He ended the day with a prayer of despair: 'My God, my God, don't leave me, keep me close to You and save me from the last act of despair!'

39

I am at the End!

A joint a la Dostoevesky.

On the evening of 23 July, Api found out that Fräulein Herzog, his surgery assistant, had been stopped in the street by the *GPU* the previous day. No one knew what had become of her. Api himself had not reported to the *GPU*, had not been officially requested to do so, but had heard it through hearsay that he needed to go. Now he tortured himself with questions. Did they arrest Fräulein Herzog because of him? What would become of his loyal assistant in the hands of these torturers? He made up his mind that he had to report to the *GPU* the very next day and try to find out where Fräulein Herzog was, why she was detained and what had happened to her. Before going to bed that night Api entered into his diary only these words: 'I am at the end!' He needed strong sleeping pills that night.

Fräulein Herzog was released the next day without harm and she had not been questioned about her employer. It all had been some sort of misunderstanding, she said. Although there seemed to be no immediate danger, Api determined to report to the *GPU* anyway, but only after he got permission from the district medical officer for his move to the three rooms in Friedenau, if they were still available. Although it was urgent to find these rooms, before making any such move Api first wanted to deliver yet another letter for us to someone who was going to Uelzen. Communication with us was his first priority. That person, whom Api did not name, told him that in a cottage in Suderburg one of the new arrivals was seriously ill. Api's worst fears seemed to have come true, but how could he reach us in the face of overwhelming outside forces? Here, he knew, was a decision of life and death, the most difficult of his life, perhaps for a reunion now or never at all. He spent the afternoon in the most terrible worries about us. It felt, he wrote, like walking close to the abyss. Nevertheless, he managed to meet the district medical officer who approved his move to Friedenau. It seemed that 24 July, my mother's birthday, had brought him a little good fortune after all.

The next morning Api's hopes were shattered again. He was told at the Housing Bureau that even in the American sector *Pgs* were not allowed to rent an apartment. They could have no more than a single room. Api felt certain that this was not the idea of the occupiers but of his 'dear compatriots', as he called his fellow Germans, thinking especially of those – and he had several in mind – who had been 'the wildest, most brutal and blinded *Heil Hitlers* right until the end'. The man in the office was sympathetic yet he could not do anything. He just concluded with an apologetic shrug: 'That's how it is. Just think, all the railroad workers have been dismissed. They were state employees and had to be members of the Party. Now they have lost their jobs. And the railroads aren't working.'

Api left in despair. He had to do something to find a way to come to Suderburg. The night before he had been tortured once again by the familiar dreams of futility and failure. However much he tried to jump on a train or steal a bike, he always was unable to reach us. By five in the afternoon Api came to a decision. Despite his nightmares he would try to leave by train or by any means he could the next morning. Thinking about the possibility of tomorrow's journey he recalled the happy anticipation he had felt in March before his last trip to Suderburg. Although he had had to spend a night waiting at the cold and drafty Lehrter station, it had not bothered him. He had been warmed by the prospect of seeing us very soon. But now there was so much greater uncertainty that stood in the way of his being able to complete the trip successfully. He did not even have an identity card and without one he could be arrested at the first control stop. He also needed a place to leave his baggage for he could no longer stay at Frau Paterek's. Poor as its content was, it was all he had.

Api spent the evening with a doctor he knew who offered to put him up for the night. During their conversation Api heard more sad news, which played into his own worst fears. Their much-valued colleague Dr Wunsch had been robbed of everything he had and then arrested. While he was preparing a field bed in the study, his host strongly advised Api against the trip at this time: 'It makes no sense to leave now, without any kind of foothold in Berlin and without even an identity card. You would never be able to come back.' Reluctantly, Api agreed. As he had feared all along, and as his dreams had told him, he had to postpone his journey to us once again, at least until he could somehow obtain those three rooms in Friedenau or find another place. It was a desperate ending to a bad month.

While Api was embroiled in these personal worries, he cherished the hope that some help would come from the international stage, that is the Potsdam Conference. From 17 July to 2 August the Allies made many vital decisions about Germany. The country's eastern border was moved westward to the Oder–Neisse line, demarcated by those two rivers. It meant a 25 per cent reduction to Germany's territory. It was further decreed that demilitarisation, de-Nazification, democratisation and restitution were to become the chief aims for Germany. The German armed forces and its entire war industry were to be abolished and all heavy industry dismantled.

Despite Api's hopes, the Potsdam Conference did not immediately lead to any improvement in living conditions for the people of Germany in general, or Berlin in particular. In fact, the medical situation there continued to worsen: especially for infants up to 3 or 4 years of age, the death rate was enormous. Api was glad every day that I was no longer in Berlin. Older people were also dying in large numbers of malnutrition and disease. For weeks on end the promised 7g of fat existed only on the cheap paper of the ration cards. Even potatoes were gone and desperate Berliners had planted potatoes in the Tiergarten. Water was still scarce and dysentery and other gastrointestinal illnesses killed close to 8,000 people that summer, and many more died of tuberculosis. During the bombing, the death rate in Berlin had been about 250 people a day; now that number had climbed to 1,000. Hospitals still had too few medications and no dietary food or strengthening nutrition whatsoever for convalescents, not even milk for pregnant and nursing mothers. Only children up to 24 months were allowed a daily 0.25l of milk.

The Potsdam Conference also brought no relief for *Pgs*. Api still could not rent his own apartment. Nevertheless, he went to the see Frau Winkler, the landlady of the place Dr Blumann had mentioned. The address was Begastrasse 10 in Friedenau, 3 miles straight south from where he had been. Although he noticed that there were no window panes left and the grey stucco was crumbling, the building was in far better shape than almost anything he had seen in Berlin Mitte. What delighted Api most was that the linden trees which lined both sides of Begastrasse were still alive, and there was a little mountain ash in the tiny green space right in front of the downstairs window.

After talking to Frau Winkler they came up with a solution to the rent problem which would help both Api and her. She would sub-let the rooms to him so that Api would have a place to stay and she some much-needed extra income. Frau Winkler noticed that Api was having a difficult time coping with everything and she exploited his desperate situation to her benefit. She charged him 120 Reichsmarks for his three rooms. The rent for her five rooms and balcony was only 152. When Api objected, she accused him of being petty. She refused to see his poverty, and insisted: 'You doctors always have mountains of money.' It must be said in her defence, and Api acknowledged this as well, that Frau Winkler's life was difficult too. She had to fight for everything all by herself. Her husband, a 55-year-old member of the *Volkssturm*, had died in the war and the Americans had requisitioned whatever good furniture and carpets she had for use in their own quarters.

The rooms also disappointed Api. The windows were broken and, as Dr Blumann had told him, so was part of one wall. It was 'a joint a la Dostoevsky'. Regardless, Api consoled himself, this would give him a foothold. The mention of Dostoevsky made him think of his beloved son who had been avidly reading the novels during his convalescence and had also recommended them to Api. When Frau Winkler revised her offer by adding that to begin with he could only have two of the three rooms, Api accepted that also. He saw no other option; it still was better than being out on the street. Frau Paterek had been most kind, but she needed her room back and, anyway, he had begun to feel like a parasite. Two rooms, he told himself, would be enough to open a surgery, even if he had to sleep in one of them. He also felt a little safer away from the Russian sector, although he worried that 'perhaps they will take me away after all! I have almost no hope.'

Mike and I visited Begastrasse 10 in 2008. The S-Bahn took us from Potsdamer Platz to the Wannsee Station Friedenau. The train went on in direction of the Grunewald, halfway to Potsdam. We crossed the square in front of the station and after a few steps came to the Dürer Platz, another little square, from where we entered Begastrasse. It was a short and quiet tree-lined street, just as Api had described it. We found No. 10 halfway down on the right side. We stood in front of the grey stucco building, which now was well taken care of. It was three stories high, with tall bay windows in the front. The front garden had a tiny patch of grass, but the mountain ash Api had enjoyed was gone.

When Api first moved to Begastrasse 10 the trains did not run, but they started soon afterwards. Having at last found a space to himself, Api immediately went to the American commandant to get permission to go to Suderburg for a visit. Permission was denied since *Pgs* were not allowed out of Berlin. Or, the official added, if a *Pg* somehow already was outside the city, he was not allowed to return either. This brought Api's expectation of a reunion with us down to zero. Once again he reproached himself for not trying to flee Berlin immediately at the end of hostilities and long before the division of the city. But, he reminded himself, going around in familiar circles in his mind, there had been so many reasons that had kept him there: his duty as a doctor, the loss of our livelihood and the great possibility that he would be captured on the way and deported.

The American commandant also changed Api's ration card back to the lowest group, known as the cemetery or death card. This meant, if you were lucky, 20g (7oz) meat, 7g (0.2oz) fat, 300g (10oz) bread, 400g (14oz) potatoes and 15g (0.5oz) sugar. On the streets starving people offered up their last possessions for any kind of food. Api could tolerate the hunger better than the pain of not being able to see us and the fear of arrest with the prospect of torture.

With this news from the commandant, Api could see no future. So, resigned, he took out his diary to tell us the names of people with whom he had deposited what little mementoes he had left. He entered the names in a framed square on the inside back cover of the green booklet so that we would be sure to notice them. Since it would be nearly impossible to get in touch with anyone in the Soviet sector and even less likely to get anything out, he listed only his newly made friends in the American sector. He left his fountain pen with Frau Paterek and his gold watch with Frau Grossmann. He also mentioned Fräulein Herzog, who had the most immediate information about him.

After that Api felt at an end. He could not read, work, lie down or sit up. On the streets he was restless and in his rooms hardly capable of concentrated thought. He noted in despair: 'I cannot even master writing halfway collectedly in this little book which I have always loved so much ... I am afraid of great physical and mental torture. And – I do not want to abandon my God.'

40

We'd be Lucky to get Ike Cleared

How can I understand the questionnaire in any other than way than as a modern attempt to make me examine my conscience?

Now that Api was installed in the American zone, he realised that it had challenges of its own. He found that the Americans were at least as dedicated to de-Nazification as the Russians had been and made life difficult for *Pgs*. Historian Giles MacDonogh notes: 'The Americans insisted that *de-Nazification* be carried out with a toughness absent from the other zones.' To begin with, everyone had to fill out a questionnaire that ran to twelve pages with 132 questions. MacDonogh goes on to say that 'it was only once the properly completed questionnaire had been returned and vetted that a German could return to normal life. Until then he was in a sort of purgatory that left him outside the law.' Americans handled almost 170,000 cases whereas the British had only 2,296. By December 1945, 90,000 Nazis were imprisoned in the American zone. As Joseph Kanon has an American officer exclaim in his novel *The Good German*, 'De-Nazification. Those guys – we'd be lucky to get Ike cleared.'

Api struggled with the questionnaire for a long time. He often felt at a loss of how to answer a question to which he saw no easy response. Yet no space, the form warned, was to be left blank. One of the questions on that list was whether you had ever hoped for German victory. How could anyone answer this truthfully? Who in any country had never hoped for their own victory? But if you said yes, what would happen? Glancing at the other questions, Api feared that his answers would not go down well with the Americans. The questionnaire seemed to make little distinction between being a Nazi and a Prussian. Api's Prussian background, to say nothing of his education at a military academy, would no doubt be held against him. Having been a member of the *Stahlhelm* put him, he feared, at further disadvantage. Even his membership in a student fraternity might come to haunt him. Api shook his head in frustration. The questioners seemed to have no idea that the Nazis had been against fraternities from the beginning and had even suspended them since 1935. Another perplexing question asked whether the bombing had affected health, work or sleep. Had these questioners never experienced a bombing raid? Then he had to list every trip abroad he had ever taken, every relative who held an office, every membership in an organisation. Perhaps, he thought, it was safer not to fill it out at all.

In 1951, six years after those questionnaires were issued, novelist Ernst von Salomon wrote a witty and insightful book about them. He used the 132 questions to examine his life, answering even supposedly simple questions with long discursive answers in a novel of over 700 pages. For example, question No. 11 asked only for the person's address, but Salomon cannot find an easy answer even to that simple enquiry since at that time his abode was 'as fleeting as the moment'. His novel shows the absurdity of this bureaucratic instrument that attempts to shove everyone into clear categories. At the same time, it offers a detailed account of the Nazi years. Going deeper, the questions serve as trigger for Salomon to probe his conscience. 'How can I,' he asks himself, 'understand the questionnaire in any other way than as a modern attempt to make me examine my conscience?' Pondering this, Salomon has one of his chief characters remark, 'Today we are all made responsible. Today we are not only asked about what we have done, but also about what we have not done.' Then again, the storyteller cannot suppress his anger at the humiliation the questioners impose on him and at the moral superiority they so easily assume, which shows little understanding of what went on during those twelve Nazi years.

I do not know whether some such thoughts also passed through Api's mind as he sat for hours in front of the questionnaire, but it is clear that for the moment he was unable to complete that document and laid it down in frustration as often as he picked it up.

41

Aborted Journeys

My God, doctor, if one always considers all and
every possibility, one gets nothing done.

Api did not give up his attempts to communicate with us,
although he had as little success with this as with the
questionnaire. On Sunday morning, 5 August, he was once
again in search of a man who, he had heard, was travelling out
of Berlin and heading for northern Germany somewhere in the proximity
of Suderburg. Api did not say who the man was or how he had heard about
him, but mentioned that he had to walk a long way from Begastrasse to
find him. When he got to the appointed address, Api was told that the man
was in church. So he walked to the nearby church and waited outside,
hoping that it was the right one. The church stood on one side of a square
surrounded by trees, but the shingles of its roof were gone and the stained-
glass windows shattered. Sitting on a bench across from the church, Api
contemplated this sight. Despite his pain, and the prospect of the damaged
church, he took in the wonder of the mild morning bathed in a soft light. He
noticed how above this ruin 'arched a sky of rare beauty, a deep blue with
white cumulus clouds'.

Just then the sounds of a well-preserved organ drifted over to him from
the church. As he sat on his bench listening intently, it felt as if he was

rising up into the heavens along with the majestic harmonies. Then the congregation, which must have been large, burst into the hymn *How shall I not be grateful to my Lord, how not praise Him.* Api listened with rapture while the organ accompanied by the human voices resounded through the open roof into the sky.

After the service was over, Api and the man somehow identified each other. Api handed his precious letter to him together with urgent entreaties to help it towards its destination. The man explained his route to the west, which he considered relatively safe and mentioned a particular spot as the best place to get across the 'green border' at the River Elbe, which was the as yet unmarked separation between East and West. Api listened carefully but did not entrust the location even to his diary.

Inspired by the stranger's initiative, Api bought a ticket for Suderburg knowing full well that a ticket was no guarantee of getting on a train. He was glad that he had been able to save enough money from his patients to be able to afford this. It felt good just holding the ticket in his hands, a palpable token of a reunion. If he could not make it all the way, he would follow the suggestion of the man and somehow get across the green border at the point he had indicated. Fräulein Herzog, who had followed Api out of Berlin Mitte hoping to work with him again, told him that if he left she wanted to come too. There was nothing and no one keeping her in Berlin.

With the train tickets in his pocket, Api joined a long line of people outside a grocery store, hoping to get some bread for the journey. Two men in line right behind him were talking about the green border, and the way out of Berlin. One of them said that he had heard that locals reported difficulties at the very place where Api had hoped to cross. 'Many already have lost their lives there and many others are still waiting, hidden in wheat fields. Both the Russians and the Brits know about this spot and watch it carefully. If you are caught, you most likely are dead.' Api had no idea how trustworthy this rumour was, but he felt as if an irony of fate had put that man in his path just at this time.

That evening Fräulein Herzog showed up at his door firmly committed to the journey and almost enthusiastic. The train was to leave at 11 p.m. The night was eerie and dark, with thunderstorms threatening all around. They debated yet again whether it was safer to leave or to stay. Api told her what he had overheard in the food line but Fräulein Herzog brushed it off as just another wild rumour. He also feared the added burden of dragging Fräulein Herzog into danger with him. Then he had to consider for the hundredth time that, even if he did get through, the British occupation authorities of Suderburg certainly would not allow him to stay in their zone. How then would he ever get back to Berlin? Fräulein Herzog could only say: 'My God, doctor, if one always considers all and every possibility, one gets nothing done.' He had to agree and yet could not make a move.

The hours went by in fruitless discussion and they did not leave. After 11 p.m. had come and gone, Api just sat there, spent. Fräulein Herzog stayed with him for the rest of the night talking to him about her home, now lost to her. Api commiserated with her, but he did not have much energy left. He was hardly able to speak, and felt that his thoughts were no longer fully under his control.

So once again Api's plan had come to nothing. August dragged on exhaustingly and hopelessly. He hardly wrote in his diary any more. The main writing he did was postcards and letters to us, in part, perhaps, to make up for his inability to leave. He not only asked travellers to take these messages with them but he also wrote to strangers in the area of Suderburg to beg them to please let his wife and daughter know that he had survived. Most of these efforts were in vain, but in my mother's box I found proof that one of these notes had been successful. I was delighted when I dug the little card out of my mother's papers and could actually read Api's plea and imagine the joy that the arrival of the card must have caused with Nyussi and my mother. On 25 August Api wrote to Herr Frohns, owner of the Frohns Hotel in Uelzen. He said that a mutual friend, Herr Gerhardt from Luisenstrasse, had given him this contact and implored Herr Frohns to forward the card or send a messenger to Suderburg telling us that he was alive and that he had moved to Begastrasse 10 in Friedenau. He also asked another favour. Would Herr Frohns allow us to give him a postcard in return? Then, when he knew of someone at his hotel who was planning to travel to Berlin or as near to Berlin as possible, would Herr Frohns hand him the card for mailing or delivery? It would be best, Api added, if the card were mailed in Berlin or if the person would deliver it to him directly. Api explained that the Wannsee train, which left from Potsdamer station and ran pretty regularly now, stopped almost immediately next to Begastrasse

10. This was a bit of an exaggeration since his rooms were two blocks from the station, but he so wanted to hear from the messenger. He concluded that whoever undertook this task would be generously rewarded for his pains.

Api did not know what else he could do. So he waited, ran mainly fruitless errands, saw a patient here and there, tried to find enough food to keep from starving and wrote more letters. But he did not touch his green diary.

On 22 August, when no patients appeared, he used the empty time to write another letter. This one must have reached us in Suderburg or perhaps Api just held on to it. Either way, sixty years later I uncovered it in my mother's lockbox and it helps to fill in the time without diary entries. Api wrote to us about his many frustrations and few small successes. At 8 a.m. that day he had reported to the magistrate of the Steglitz-Friedenau district to try yet again to obtain permission to travel. I do not understand the bureaucratic jungle of that time, but this time he was given a long form to fill out. In it he stated that his reasons for seeking the travel permission were to secure his medical instruments out of Berlin and to visit sick relatives. He hoped that would do.

The form by itself was not enough. He still needed to complete the American twelve-page questionnaire. In addition to that difficult task he had to provide an affidavit from the person who was in charge of the apartment building where he lived. In an attempt to organise the population, a foreman had been assigned to each building in the city. Their job was to watch the house and its lodgers, who in turn had to address any reports or concerns to the foreman. It was a system that facilitated spying and denunciations of all sorts. The Nazis had used something very similar when they put block wardens in charge of every city block. Since Api was not yet known at his new address and was only sub-letting anyway, he assumed that he had to obtain this declaration from the foreman at Luisenstrasse 41. Frau Gertrud Albrecht, who had been the building manager for all the years he had lived there, was no longer in charge, and a stranger had taken her place. So he probably would run into the same obstacle again. He was after all a *Pg*, a creature without rights and without protection for whom nothing could or should be done.

There was yet another requirement before the authorities would consider the travel permission. Api had to get approval from the Soviet commanding officer in charge of Luisenstrasse. This especially frightened Api. Would he not attract the attention of the *GPU*, the Soviet secret police, especially since they may have been looking for him anyway? Although he could not imagine any possible denunciation against him, he feared the *GPU* and its unpredictable procedures. And perhaps, he wondered, it was true that his military discharge signed by Professor Sauerbruch back in May was invalid after all. There had been rumours that Professor Sauerbruch had been dismissed and all his decisions had been rescinded. But no one knew anything definite.

It seems likely to me today that these rumours were related to Sauerbruch's ambivalent role during the Nazi regime, which was typical of many people in high places who were not outright Nazis. Professor Sauerbruch, in fact, was not dismissed from the Health Bureau until 12 October 1945, when he was charged with having contributed to the reputation of the Nazi regime, and he was almost immediately reinstated at the Charité. But in August Api just had rumours, not knowing what to believe, so that the validity of his military discharge continued to worry him. With all these hurdles, it seemed that Api's only options were, as they had always been, to attempt a secret crossing at the green border or stay in Berlin.

42

Have I a Right?

A heart, even if it lies completely in ruins, keeps on
hoping and no experience can teach it otherwise.

As still no patients appeared, the letter to us grew longer and longer. Api voiced yet again his anxiety about our welfare and his yearning to be with us. Above all he felt a deep sense of responsibility that it was up to him to look after us, a responsibility he could not abandon just because he felt at an end. 'Have I a right,' he asked, 'to throw down everything here and destroy our hope for a possibly secure future?' For once he left Berlin, it was pretty well certain that he would not be allowed to return to work there. At the worst he could be arrested and sent away.

The starvation diet – weeks without meat, fresh vegetables or fat – had seriously reduced Api's energy. He had become skeletal. He could not even look into the mirror any more when he washed himself. His scrawny arms and legs were as wrinkled as his mother's had been just before her death. Yet, he felt, despite everything, 'a heart, even if it lies completely in ruins, keeps on hoping and no experience can teach it otherwise'. His will to live was driven by the prospect of a reunion. He wrote:

If only all this would be nothing more than bad memories and the most terrible experiences part of the past, it then would lose its bitterness and unbearable pain ... Oh, once more with you! But if God should decree differently, then you know from my unvarnished accounts of my suffering how much I needed rest, how much I loved you, and hopefully you would find peace in the thought that it was God's will.

By now Api had filled two pages with his small rounded script, with which he could cram forty-five lines on a page. He felt a little better for having told us all about his worries and ended with sending his prayers and love, folded the paper, addressed it and crept into bed.

Two days later, on 24 August, Api wrote again: another long letter that spilled over into the next day. In it he continued to air the tormenting dilemmas he had already confided to the diary. Had he done the right thing to leave their home on Luisenstrasse? He had to admit that at his new place on Begastrasse he also saw only few patients. In fact, just then his surgery was empty again. Yet he hoped that here at least was the possibility of a new start because the area was inhabited. Once he became known his practice would prosper again. In all his quandaries Api never forgot that he was by no means without friends and acquaintances who supported him physically as well as emotionally. In fact, he knew and told us that he was better off than many others in Berlin. He began to list all the people who had helped him these past months and he was filled with gratitude. Although Api did not acknowledge this, I am struck that all of them were women.

He first thought of Frau Grossmann. She regularly invited him to her place and offered both food and companionship. Frau Paterek from the Housing Bureau was another person who helped out. She had given Api the job of administering typhoid inoculations out of her home, which earned him a little money. Frau Paterek also had put him up when he had nowhere to go and she, too, occasionally invited him to a meal.

Next, Api thought of Fräulein Herzog, his assistant. Although they hardly had any patients, Fräulein Herzog was always there to support him. Api was much moved by her care. Whenever possible she cooked a warm meal for him on his one electric burner and she also tried to cheer him up, although she herself had lost everything and was all alone in the world. He asked us: 'If I should not be able to cope, thank her at least in your hearts if you cannot do it otherwise.'

Api also thought gratefully of the patients who shared with him the little they had, bringing him a jar of home-made jam or a pudding and making sure his surgery was never without flowers. Finally his thoughts turned to the deaconesses who had befriended him, both here and in Berlin Mitte. They allowed him to share in their company and he felt strengthened by their charity and their faith.

These kind women comforted Api, and he could not have managed without their help, but he concluded that nothing could wipe away his despair or overcome his exhaustion of body and mind. His life had shrunk down to one dominant emotion, anxiety, which made it impossible for him to decide anything. One moment he would make up his mind to leave and so he would start the cumbersome process of applying for the various permissions; and the very next moment he would have to expend an equal amount of energy to undo everything.

At the end of August Api made one other attempt to get out of Berlin. His friends, the two deaconesses, had introduced him to a Herr Reese who was leaving for Uelzen, so that Api could give him a letter to take along for Suderburg. Instead of just handing over another letter to a stranger as he had done so often before, Api decided on the spur of the moment to join the man on his trip. He knew that he would not be able to go on his own, and here was a companion who travelled essentially the same way. Before leaving for the station on 28 August, Api just jotted three words in his diary: 'Plan for departure.' Then he packed his rucksack and started the long trek to the East station. He joined his fellow traveller and they waited a long time on the crowded platform. When the train finally pulled into the station it was so full, Api wrote later in a letter, that not even a cigar box would have fitted in. A few desperate or adventurous men even clung to the steps and the roof. It was hopeless to get on. The man told Api that he himself would try again the next day, but this time he would go early to Anhalter station, south of Potsdamer Platz. Api thought fleetingly of the many times he had taken Nyussi and the children to that station with its huge domed hall for their journey to Hungary. Then he heard the man's further explanation that it was Berlin's busiest station right now with more trains leaving from there every day. They would have a much better chance of getting on to one of them. It is true, the man admitted, that from Anhalter station they would have to follow a circuitous route, first to Halle and then make their way by various other connections west to Uelzen, but it would be better than waiting here for a direct train and never being able to squeeze on. He invited Api to come along.

Api watched the man leave, admiring how easily he made his decisions. Api, for his part, was once again at a loss of what to do. It was afternoon by now and he had already walked more than 5 miles from Begastrasse to the East station carrying his rucksack on his back. There were still hours of daylight ahead and he felt he had to do something with this day. So he made up his mind to walk a little further to Lehrter station, just west of the Charité. It would be less than 2 miles from where he was. He wanted to check whether he could find a more direct train from there than the roundabout route via Anhalter station. But when Api reached Lehrter station, he saw signs posted everywhere telling him that as of now and until further notice travel to the British zone was forbidden. So there would be no trains at all to Uelzen from there. He had to turn around and start the long hike back to Friedenau, having accomplished nothing. When he got home, he dumped his rucksack without unpacking it, and wrote in his diary: 'Missed departure.' He had no strength to say anything more.

Api was still tired out the day after that failed trip, exhausted from the disappointment as much as from the long hike. He stayed home and began another letter, feeling that he had to explain to us, and perhaps to himself, why he had not left after all. Underlying all the arguments why he was not on the train ran a refrain of self-reproach and shame for his weakness.

That same day the Russian sector announced that all members of the military from lieutenant on up, as well as all *Pgs*, had to report for registration to the Russian commander by 25 September. As a result, Api felt certain that staying in place would be the greatest stupidity of his life and yet still all the familiar counter-arguments kept crowding in on him. Feeling his brain spin in a vortex around the same questions, he felt that it was all too much for him to cope with all alone. Whenever he had faced difficulties before, Nyussi had been at his side with her love, her strength and her courage, and he could listen to her always level-headed and unsentimental advice. Now, however, he seriously doubted whether he would be able to handle anything alone. Even as he was writing to her, he said that he was so distraught that he had to jump up, rip the spectacles off his nose, stamp his foot and curse himself for a coward. After he had finished the letter, he reached for his green booklet and quickly scribbled his last entry of the month: 'If only one could at last give up!! God be with you.'

43

Listen to the Grasshoppers

If all people would become God's collaborators ...
all this terrible misery could be mastered – one might
say in a moment.

The beginning of September was no better than the end of August had been. In one sense it was even worse because autumn inexorably came closer, soon to be followed by winter. It was not a happy prospect in Api's ground-floor rooms without a stove and with only cardboard in the windows.

On Sunday 9 September Api started another diary, perhaps because he had given the first into safekeeping. The new diary was outwardly identical to the previous one: a 3.5in x 5.5in booklet with a sturdy cover of green cloth and 'AGENDA' stencilled in gold at the top. The beginning pages had lists of patients and their payments, dating back to earlier years. The amounts Api had pencilled in varied between 3 and 10 Reichsmarks with a very occasional 20 or 30 Reichsmarks, but all of them were sums that now seemed to him like a miracle.

As Api sat down to write in this diary, the first word that came to his mind was simply 'Destruction', but then he recalled Superintendent Pfeifer's sermon he had just heard that morning. Its theme was: 'If all people would become God's collaborators, if everyone would administer our earthly goods with the love taught and lived by our Lord Jesus Christ, all this terrible misery could be mastered – one might say in a moment.' Api had listened attentively to these words, which echoed his own sentiments and his daily devotional readings. The sermon had been followed by a choir with a violin solo. Although the violinist interested Api and he listened closely to the beautiful and technically accomplished performance, he did not mention the piece he was playing. Instead he noted that even while listening to the beautiful harmonies, he had to fight with himself not to be overwhelmed by anger and rebellion. This was the first time in his fearful and lonely existence that anger and bitterness became dominant. Api had been anxious and even desperate before, but not angry or bitter. It was probably a sign that he was losing all hope for the future. He was afraid to be overwhelmed by these violent emotions because they stood in the way of his faith and he so wanted to maintain a Christian disposition. But with each passing day that was getting more difficult.

After church Api cycled the short distance to Frau Paterek to administer typhoid inoculations. A typhoid epidemic continued to be a serious threat and the Allies had ordered inoculations for the population. Api found several people at her home, which earned him a little money, but, as had become his habit, he charged far less than the regular amount for the inoculations. He did it gladly but at the same time he was a little annoyed with himself. He needed the money to fix up his rooms, find moulding to cover the cracks in the wallboard and, above all, replace the cardboard in his windows with real panes of glass. Frau Paterek, however, rewarded his generosity by inviting him to lunch. It was his first warm food in days.

Inevitably the conversation focused on the current situation. Someone mentioned that he had heard that all *Pgs* were supposed to be transported to work camps. 'From the Russian zone, he said, they are to be sent to Russia, and from the Anglo-American zone to France or Belgium.' Hearing this, Api only thought to himself, 'as is God's will, one cannot evade it'. He had become almost inured to the constant fear.

Nevertheless, Api continued to be haunted by his *Pg* status. He thought that the unending smear propaganda had accelerated the hatred of *Pgs* into a psychosis – if only, he admitted to himself, with the non-thinking population. Yet because he was a *Pg* his every move was blocked. He was unable to establish himself, to rent an apartment or to obtain permission to travel. He had the lowest ration card and there was no hope of getting a telephone connection for his surgery room, and, perhaps worst of all, his outcast status broke him down. He himself began to feel like a second-class citizen, even a criminal, hardly human. On occasion his spirit revolted against this and he asked himself when had he ever hurt anyone politically in the slightest? What had he done politically at all? However much Api examined his life, he was certain that his boundless happiness:

did not happen at the expense of any other human being whatsoever ... And yet the propaganda creates a veritable psychosis of hatred against people who had the misfortune to be inscribed, a psychosis which claims almost every one without exception who, without having been *Pgs*, agitated infinitely more wildly for the aims of national socialist Germany, yes, even abused me as a poor member of the Party if I dared call things by their right names and predict our fate.

The question of political responsibility was, of course, the point with which the Allies vehemently disagreed with most Germans, and which we still debate today. Were all Germans guilty of the atrocities committed in their name by the Hitler regime? If so, to what degree? Is Api's defence that he had not done anything politically a valid argument, or do we not think today that doing nothing carries with it a responsibility, especially since he had to have been a daily witness to persecution? Do we then have to find Germans collectively guilty, and perhaps people of my grandfather's class – educated, well-to-do members of the upper-middle class – most of all? It is a dilemma with which I continue to struggle. However, today I can debate it all at leisure and in peace, far from the world in which Api barely survived. He had no such luxury and so, perhaps, put any thoughts of guilt and responsibility out of his mind.

Alone in his rooms at night, Api fell into despair. He even played with the idea of giving up and selling his instruments 'in exchange for no matter how primitive and uncreative a line of work'. Labourers were needed everywhere but, of course, Api was just fantasising. He had little, if any, such skills – had not even been able to fix a light or a dripping tap in their home before the war. He was also well aware that the German Reichsmark was not worth much at this point and whatever little value it had left was unstable. Therefore, selling precious medical equipment in exchange for possibly worthless Reichsmarks made little economic sense. Api realised that he was just desperately dreaming of ways to survive.

Having heard that the entire town of Oranienburg just north of Berlin was under quarantine because of the typhoid epidemic, Api at last gave himself an inoculation. It resulted in days of misery with fever and chills. Despite that, he kept his surgery open and a few eye patients straggled in to be treated. The week passed in a sad and largely lonely routine and on Saturday evening, 15 September, he sought refuge in the company of a friend, the deaconess Sister Minna. I do not know how they were acquainted except that there must have been close associations between all the deaconesses in Berlin who travelled to clinics and hospitals where they were needed.

Sister Minna's mother house was at Birkbuxstrasse 30 in Berlin Lichterfelde, only 5km (just over 3 miles) south of where Api lived. When he got there another old friend, Sister Ottilie, joined them as well. Sister Ottilie originally came from Tieckstrasse 17, the mother house of deaconesses Baesler and Briese in Berlin Mitte.

Sister Minna's mother house had a large walled garden and Api was allowed to pick the seeds out of sunflowers that were ripening by the garden wall. He happily chewed them for a little fat. Then they all went inside. After praying together, the sisters fed him coffee and bread with raspberry jam and built him up with their religious, yet at the same time worldly wise, conversation. On leaving, they presented him with a heavy little cardboard case. When he opened the lid to peek inside, he found two heads of cauliflower, fourteen tomatoes, four pears and, well aware of his love of sweets, a piece of cake. He thanked the generous sisters with tears in his eyes.

As he stepped outside Api noticed that it was beginning to get dark, another sign of the approaching winter. He hoped that he would be in time to catch the last train, which would save him about half the distance of his hike. But when he reached the station the train was just pulling out, which he thought was typical of the bad luck that seemed to follow him everywhere. In a dejected mood he trudged on through the darkening and empty streets.

Carrying his heavy but invaluable burden, Api listened to the grasshoppers. Their whirring and chirping drew his thoughts back to when he was a child in Marienwerder. He remembered how often, when his homework was done, he had cycled past fields of rye, oats and potatoes to get to his favourite spots near the wide Weichsel River. He had explored the marshy meadows and little ponds ringed by hawthorns, sloes and alders, the homes of turtles and woodcocks. He had crept silently up to a pond to observe the long-legged water birds. He also noticed the curlews with beaks almost as long as their bodies, squat plovers with their dramatic black neck stripes and elegant sandpipers in their black and brown coats. In winter the shallow ponds froze early and were excellent for skating.

It was summer holidays Api liked best, however, when he could be outside all day. Above all, he loved the fat green grasshoppers as they jumped and hummed all over the sunny meadows. He thought of them as the friends of his youth. I share Api's love of grasshoppers, which were also abundant in the meadow outside the home where I lived with my grandparents. I loved to lie in the grass to watch them whirring around me. If I was very still a few settled on my hands and arms, and I felt tickled by their scratchy little legs. Listening to them now, however, Api noticed that these city grasshoppers already 'chirped autumnally voiceless'. This finally brought him back to the present. He thought with dread of the winter to come. The cardboard in his windows would not keep out the cold. On chilly days the wind already was whistling through the cracks in the floorboards and moulding.

At home, sitting down with the companionship of his diary, Api recalled the scene of his walk and the beauty of the evening mellowed him. 'The moon was behind clouds, the darkness was penumbrous, a warm September evening rested silently over holy, indelible, but already oh so distant memories!' He was saddened that even memories of his happy childhood, which before always had been a source of strength, had begun to fade. It all seemed so far away and unrecoverable. Before going to sleep, Api knocked on his landlady's door and shared with her some of his gifts from Sister Ottilie. She accepted sourly and his hope that their relationship would become warmer and more open was dashed right away.

221

44

A Bad Christian

Some mornings I am shaken by spasms of horror and I have to fight with an iron will that I don't give up everything in despair, crawl under my sheets and wait for the end – or bring it about!

On Sunday the fever from the inoculation had lessened and Api started the day with a complete wash. The cold water did him good. He had always believed in the recuperative power of cold showers. When I lived with my grandparents in Bevensen in the early 1950s he often insisted I take a cold shower in the morning, to which I submitted with shrieks of terror and delight. We were one of few only a German families at that time who had a shower at all, since most people had only bathtubs. Our shower was a large room tiled in a cream colour, in which I could jump about, alternating between letting the cold water hit me and avoiding it. Api's predilection for showers, especially cold ones, has not stuck with me and today I prefer hot and lazy baths.

Despite his cold-water wash, Api was depressed. As it had been in his attic room, mornings were his worst times. He often now lay awake for a long time before he plucked up courage to get out of bed. Tormented by loneliness and anxiety, he was tempted just to hide away under the covers. There was so much that he feared. He was afraid:

that no patients will come, that something will happen politically, that I cannot bear up economically, that my desperate longing makes me do something stupid, that the days and weeks go by too slowly, that perhaps a reunion will no longer be granted us and if so – how terribly hopeless it will be, that perhaps you are not all alive any more or are sick, that I will not be able to make my apartment liveable for the winter, that all my errands in that regard will fail where others succeed!

Api felt guilty that he began the day as a bad Christian with this panic-like fear. Even prayer did not help, or rather he could not pray at all. Instead his thoughts strayed back to the past. He calculated that during the last twenty years he had put in at least 43,500 hours of work and now everything had come down to naught. He thought of all those who once had been part of his life and now were gone: his mother and father, his son, his son-in-law. Then for moments it seemed as if his son was with him again, and yet he was not dreaming. Or perhaps it was because, he speculated, he already belonged more to those who were dead than to the living. He was beginning to feel dead inside. It was getting harder to remember the joy of the brisk autumn holidays in the Riesengebirge with Nyussi, where in the evenings they sat together to play a game chess, each with a glass of red wine, and he enjoyed his nightly cigar. It all seemed so irretrievably lost. He could no longer muster the discipline and control which had been his protection against attacks of anxiety and gloom. Now he was plagued by foreboding whether his mind would hold out.

As he began to lose himself in dreams of Nyussi and the harmony they had enjoyed, he told himself that he had to keep away from thoughts about how life had been and how it never would be again. For whenever such memories ambushed him they knocked him down and made him bitter, and he was ashamed that in this way he was railing against God. That, he told himself, was unworthy of a Christian. 'Only not judge and reckon with God, and say that everything is blind chance after all. I am certain that it is God's will, even if I cannot understand it and that somehow it must work toward our benefit.' He remembered the hymn whose verses he often read at night, *A Christian cannot be without a cross*. He tried to console himself with the thought that 'the larger the cross, the more beautiful the reward'.

He also knew that he was part of a large community that was living in similar misery.

However, the futile errands with which he struggled day by day kept him down. He tried in vain to move up to a better category of ration card. He kept showing up at the Housing Bureau in search of more permanent accommodation which, likewise, came to nothing. Even his application at the district office for basic necessities, including undergarments, was not successful. In addition to these official visits, Api also was constantly in search of a glazier for his windows, but was told no again and again. He knew that if he had cigarettes or alcohol with which to bribe the men he would have better luck. Despite running around much of the day, he wished for more work and less time to feel his loneliness. He still did regular inoculations at Frau Paterek's and read his medical text, but it was not enough to support him, much less make a livelihood.

Each morning Api forced himself to break through that cycle of fears, memories and speculations. 'Sometimes I think my heart simply stops in a physical spasm and strain.' However, after he had prepared his flour soup on his burner he felt a little stronger, ready to clean his rooms and make the bed so that everything was ready for any patients that might come. These unfamiliar household chores were to him a pleasant distraction and for a little while they kept him from facing the more problematic tasks of his existence. But not for long:

> When I crawl into the bathroom, and shave myself, chilled, in the half light, then cook my flour soup and in between clean my boots, make the bed and eat my breakfast while cleaning up, watch how the time for my urgent agenda increasingly shrivels up, until one thing after another has to be given up, how one or the other errand which I hastily try to accomplish, is always, always futile, and the threat of the cold and the postponement of other things becomes ever greater: I am in the grips of the whole misery of mankind!

45

A Little Closer to Thee

Our true home after all is the heavenly eternity –
without separation, without tears, without disquiet,
Angst, and pains of the heart!

Api was standing by the open window on the evening of Wednesday 19 September, listening once again to his friends the grasshoppers:

Silently and big rises the almost full slice of the moon above the light fog across the meadows. The edge of the big city with a few lit windows in the distance ... Grasshoppers sing to me of my own youth which was infinitely joyful despite rather straightened circumstances.

As it was getting dark, he noticed fireworks in the south-east from the direction of Treptow. He was amazed how soon Berlin revived the Wednesday tradition of 'Treptow in Flames', a weekly firework show near the River Spree, which had been popular before the war. When my mother and uncle were small, Api had occasionally taken them there to watch the fireworks. Afterwards he had treated them to cakes and soda in one of the many coffee houses along the river, 'very big happiness'.

On Sunday 23 September Api cherished the illusion that he had come a little closer to us. Berlin switched to winter time by moving clocks back an hour. Now perhaps, he thought, our 'oh so terribly and painfully separate life can at least run somewhat more parallel time wise'. But the time switch also reminded him that autumn was here and he prepared himself by blocking his windows more securely with pieces of cardboard. The leaves had already begun to fall, and the mountain ash outside his window was resplendent with bunches of bright red berries. He had gathered berries just like these for Nyussi in Dahlem at the beginning of their marriage when she had come home after an illness. How painfully different it all was now where he sat alone in the cold and cheerless rooms with only his sad thoughts for company.

The following Monday Api had to report yet again for registration as a *Pg*, this time in the district of Friedenau where he now lived. When he got there he was told that as officer of the former Wehrmacht he also needed to be fingerprinted. It made him feel even more like a criminal, now also with a criminal record. Yet he knew himself to be lucky compared to many medical officers of higher rank who had been captured and imprisoned. He had heard that this was true of Dr Pellnitz, who had been in charge of all the military clinics in the inner city. Also Dr Kleberger, who had given Api so much trouble when he dismissed him in May. They were both still in captivity, and yet neither had been a member of the Nazi Party. Api did not know that these men were the victims of a general policy pursued by the Allies. As Giles MacDonogh, a historian of the immediate post-war era, says: 'The Allies were obsessed with the need to stamp out "militarism", and any connection with the armed forces was held against the supplicant.'

That evening Frau Grossmann invited Api to a warm dinner of vegetable soup and apple biscuits. He set out to walk the short distance to her place, which took him past a small park where he spotted a little girl my age happily chatting with her mother. It was a sight that moved him to tears. Seeing a 3-year-old girl who reminded him of me was always one of the hardest things for him to bear. Api recovered himself enough to greet Frau Grossmann with a smile. While she was busy in the kitchen, he went over to the window and looked out on her little street, the Riemenschneiderweg. It faced a park and allotment gardens, small parcels of public land that were given to apartment dwellers so they could enjoy their own gardens. Some had built little huts on their land where they stored their equipment or even spent the night. But now the gardens had turned into a field grown wild. To the left, Api noticed a group of poplars which were crowded with hundreds of starlings. He watched the starlings as intently as he had observed the swallows from his attic. When they all flew off together with a thunderous whirring of wings, he envied them. They were free!

I was surprised to find the location of Frau Grossmann's apartment on Riemenschneiderweg almost unchanged from Api's descriptions. When Mike and I took the short walk from Begastrasse to Riemenschneiderweg, going past the small park where Api had seen the little girl, we saw a row of modest one-storey houses that looked out on a field of allotment gardens, which now, however, were once again neatly tended. The little street had the feel of a country lane more than a city street, quite different from the nearby urban apartments on Begastrasse.

Starting 26 September, Api's practice began to pick up and there was hardly a day without at least one patient. It was also getting autumnally cold, his rooms were chilly and he still could not get window panes. On 27 September he managed to obtain curtains for two of his windows, which at least hid the cardboard. It was such a little thing, but in his circumstances it pleased him greatly and made him proud. Perhaps, he thought with pleasure, it was another tiny step toward having a home again.

As soon as he had fastened the curtains to the cardboard, a patient showed up. While Api treated him, the man told him the latest news. He had heard that any former resident of Berlin who wished to return to the city could do so until the end of the month. Api wondered whether we had already left Suderburg and were on our way back to Berlin. Although he would have liked nothing better than to be with us, he was not sure whether it would work. There was hardly room for us to stay with him and he still had no firm prospects of making a living. The whole idea might also only be another rumour – Api felt frustrated never to have definite information and always be victim to gossip.

When he was alone again, Api hoped and prayed that he would have the strength to provide for us eventually despite his mental and, yes, often even spiritual exhaustion. If only his physical condition would not deteriorate further. He was suffering from a number of potentially serious ailments: edemas around his ankles, numbness in his fingers which meant circulation problems, open wounds on his shins and constant bladder pain. 'I am not good for much anymore,' he wrote in his diary with shaky fingers; but then he added: 'My handwriting, however, only is bad because I am cold.' The temperature in his rooms had dropped below 10°C (50°F), and he had written the entry from his bed.

On Friday night Api went to a talk on 'Tolstoy's Christianity' given by Superintendent Pfeifer. On his way there he heard a man shouting for help but could not find him. During the talk he kept thinking about the man and what might have happened to him, and whether anyone had been able to come to his aid.

Saturday 29 September was a nostalgia-laden day. It was the wedding anniversary of my grandparents in 1919 and my parents in 1941. When Api woke up, his left ear rang strongly, which in popular superstition meant that someone was thinking of him. He imagined that we were also rising about this time and sending our love, yet if we had not received any of his many letters and postcards we could not even know whether he was still alive. The morning was cold and bleak, the sun without any warmth, just like his life. He was chilly inside and out.

At lunchtime he saw a few patients. Among them was the man whose screams he had heard the night before, who came to get new glasses. He told Api that last night some drunken Americans had seized and beaten him. They had taken his bicycle, his briefcase and even his spectacles. Api was shocked to discover that Berliners were not safe even in the American sector.

In the afternoon, from 4 to 7 p.m., he was back at Frau Paterek's administering more typhoid inoculations. From there he walked about 1km south to Steglitz station for another of his errands. It was beginning to get dark. As he looked up at the sky, he noted that 'between night-dark clouds like huge balls, the stars were shining from an unreachable distance, cold but clear, as if they did not see any kind of suffering on earth'. By 8 p.m. Api was home in his cold rooms. His first instinct was simply to crawl into bed, but then he thought, 'no, I must try to give this day a small festive appearance'. He still had a bit of flour, as well as one pear left over from the gift of the deaconess. So he baked pear dumplings and flour cookies directly on his burner. He had no fat and no sugar, but it was the best he could do. His wedding anniversary always had been such a special day, but now his heart was full of bitterness and pain.

Although life was better here than in the Soviet sector, the man he had treated made Api aware that the streets were dangerous here, too, and American soldiers also could go on a rampage when they were drunk. A few days after that incident another group of American soldiers, who probably had had too much to drink, broke off the black-and-white enamelled sign for Api's surgery, which he had taken from Luisenstrasse, and threw stones at the house. The following night, they knocked down and robbed a fellow lodger, right in front of the house.

The last day of September was a Sunday, which was always a somewhat calming holiday for Api. He especially enjoyed that day's sermon under the title 'We are God's co-workers'. This was, it seems, Superintendent Pfeifer's favourite theme; his attempt to explain the horrors of the past and at the same time hold out the prospect of a better future. He said that it was not God's fault but that of man if His magnificent world had become so miserable. 'All of us, and not only our own people, had no longer been co-workers of God but of the devil. Instead of using all the treasures of His wonderful earth for love, we had perverted everything to hate and murder and war.' Walking home, Api thought idly but happily that the same autumn sky arched above him and us. He made himself a lunch of *Schustertunke*, potatoes and brown sauce. During his dinner Api recalled the sermon and the hope it held for a better future if men were to become co-workers of God.

On the first day of October, Api still thought back to the sermon of the day before. Inspired by the pastor's words, he sat down at his table and wrote about the need for mutual love:

> Pray and be strong in hope and, if that is no longer possible, in the love among you and among all people! If love once again dwells in all human hearts then also will the life on God's wonderful earth again become not only bearable but beautiful. Our true home after all is the heavenly eternity – without separation, without tears, without disquiet, *Angst*, and pains of the heart!

Just the act of writing gave him a little courage and he decided that it was time to move the furniture he had stored at the Westend Hospital to his rooms in Begastrasse. A dining room set was hardly useful to him right now, nor was there much space for it, but it was the only possession he had left and he wanted to have it with him. He would be able to accommodate it better once he had the additional room he had been promised in his sublet. The landlady, however, had given no sign of relinquishing that room. So Api decided to broach the matter with her once more. He hesitantly knocked at her door. He was always afraid to confront her, because she was so very harsh and unfriendly, and indeed she opened her door with a grim face. When Api mentioned the furniture, she responded that under no circumstances would she allow that stuff to come here. After a heated discussion Api agreed, for the sake of peace, to pay 140 Reichsmarks instead of the original 120 for three rooms, even though the landlady even now was not making a move to release the third room. She knew she could get away with this because he was a *Pg* who was not supposed to have an apartment.

The argument had exhausted what little energy Api had left and it had achieved worse than nothing. He had to pay 20 Reichsmarks more than before with as little hope as ever of obtaining that third room. Cold, hunger and the stress of this futile confrontation made him almost collapse. He hurried back into his rooms and broke down on a chair. He was afraid he would faint if he got up and even had to hold on to the chair for fear of falling to the floor. It was another low point in his existence and he wondered how many more he could endure. Little did he know that his luck was about to change.

46

Deus ex Machina

Unimaginable Joy!

Three days later, on Thursday 4 October, when he least expected it, Api's fortunes changed all at once. That day the postman handed him a postcard. With a pounding heart he recognised Nyussi's and my mother's handwriting. The card was dated 18 September. Although it had taken sixteen days to arrive, it was almost a miracle that it had found its way to him since he had moved to a new place in a different sector of Berlin. He read and re-read the few words and from then on kept it close to his heart at all times. He treasured Nyussi's confidence and trust that they would manage somehow if only he were with them, but the line that echoed in his mind from then on was written by my always shrewd mother. In order not to give anything away to the censor she had written: 'Do you already know that Api certainly will come?' Surely, he thought, this was a cleverly disguised request for him to come to them? It gave him a new impetus to find a way.

It was with a lighter step that Api went out to do inoculations that day, thanking God that he had heard from us and that we were well. On his return he found red cabbage, tomatoes, his laundry and a few tobacco leaves together with a bunch of dahlias, lovingly left by Sister Ottilie. It was like Superintendent Pfeifer's sermon fulfilled, granting him the joy to experience the love of his fellow men.

During the following days Api spent many hours working with renewed energy on that frustrating American questionnaire. He needed to submit it to the American administration and it had to be approved before he could get permission to leave. Now, however, he went about his work buoyed up by the postcard in his breast pocket and full of dreams of a reunion. His practice picked up at the same time. Sometimes a patient even had to wait before he could get to him. Even his application for undergarments was granted at this time! And he found an electrician who fixed his little cooker, which had given out a few days earlier.

The weather also corresponded to Api's good mood. After the earlier cold spell, it had warmed up again and Wednesday 10 October turned out to be a beautiful day. Api could once more find words to describe nature and his state of mind:

> My only ones, a fall day of rare beauty and mild serenity lies over the wilting leaves and the last colourful blossoms. Once again a warming sun sends its golden rays across the coloured leaves of the trees which silently nod their heads in a light wind from the east as if they were in complete agreement and content with all that has happened and is happening and will happen in their lives, also with the fact that they now have to take leave of this summer existence. Oh, if I could only bring myself to attain such calm composure!

The warmer days made Api's rooms more liveable. A thrush even sang again outside his window and the sparrows whistled a tune which was better than their wintry 'cheep, cheep'.

On that day, 10 October, it was exactly half a year since Api had separated from us, a length of time we could never have anticipated in the slightest. Since the arrival of the postcard, however, he lived under the spell of my mother's words. He needed to find a way! Still, he could not relinquish this last foothold on the future, especially now that patients were beginning to seek him out. He saw no other place where he had as good a chance to start afresh as here. The journey to Suderburg was also by no means certain. Berlin was full of so many contradictory rumours about the chances of getting out of the city and across the green border. Even if he managed the journey without problems, what use would it be? Without permission to relocate he would not be allowed to stay and work in the British zone of Suderburg and he would have given up the last refuge they had in Berlin. Perhaps, he worried, it would come to that in any case and then all the pain of the last six months would have been for naught. Then again, he answered himself, it was impossible to know what lay ahead, or whether all his work so far to establish a new life had been futile. All he could do was make as good an attempt as he possibly could, no matter how poor and precarious.

Api also had responsibilities as a doctor that kept him in Berlin. He was scheduled to do public inoculations until 26 October. The typhoid epidemic was still raging; he saw such a dreadful amount of dying and no end to it. Typhus was by no means the only killer, either: people died of pneumonia, infections of all sorts and malnutrition. Recently he had treated a patient suspected of meningitis whom another doctor had been afraid to touch. Yet in order to be able to examine him he bent closely over the sick, almost delirious, young man, feeling his breath on his face.

October turned out to be a month of wonderful, totally unexpected gifts in the form of postcards. Out of the blue on Thursday 11 October another postcard arrived. This one was from a Herr Blomerius of Speerweg 26 in Frohnau in the north of Berlin. Api read it with amazement:

> Your relatives in Suderburg are waiting for you with longing. In case you intend to go there, I ask you to get in touch with me still this week. With cordial greetings, Blomerius.

Api's heart sang and rang at the prospect of the so long and so desperately awaited reunion, which now, all of a sudden, seemed to become a reality. He had dreamt about this for so long, imagined the scene so often and tried to find a way. Now it fell into his lap without his doing anything.

The sudden arrival of Herr Blomerius' card makes me think about the often despised and parodied 'Deus ex Machina', 'God out of a machine'. A dramatic effect which has been used from Greek to modern drama, it is the unexpected resolution of a dramatic plot, a sudden rescue which in earlier times often literally fell out of the sky from a contraption above the stage

233

and, therefore, was called the 'God out of a machine'. Now I speculated that the device may have more reality than I had previously imagined. Herr Blomerius – the name itself sounded strange and unreal to me – whose identity I have not been able to discover anything about, remains just such an unexpected *Deus ex Machina*. In a less fanciful mood, however, I suspected that there was a more realistic explanation. Blomerius probably was a medical colleague, especially since I found out that there was a large hospital on Speerweg in Frohnau from where he had written. But why he wrote to Api at this point, how he knew where to find him and how he knew about us in Suderburg still remains a mystery.

Api wrote that he visited Herr Blomerius at 6 a.m. the next day, although I cannot imagine how he covered the great distance between Friedenau in the south-west and Frohnau far in the north of Berlin so early in the morning, or what Herr Blomerius thought of his dawn arrival. The only way he could have managed it is by *Schnellbahn*, which must have been running again. When Api got there, his dreams indeed came true. Herr Blomerius told him:

> I can help you obtain permission from the physicians' organization so that you can leave Berlin. I can further arrange for permission from the British authorities, which you will need since Suderburg is in the British sector. It can all be arranged and you should be on your way soon.

Api was overwhelmed. He rushed back to Friedenau as fast as he could to pack his rucksack and get ready so that there would not be a moment's delay once the permissions came through. He was still afraid of the journey and had not lost his anxiety that he was always making a wrong move. At the same time, he felt a new strength and confidence surge up in him. For the first time in months he could cherish a hope that was not based on mere fantasies. Once the little he had was safely packed Api sat down, opened his diary – his companion through all these months – and wrote in it for the last time, giving voice to a hope that still was a little tentative: 'Perhaps even such a poor awkward bird as I can manage to get through this? ... God bless my plan and protect you and me in His mercy.'

47

Zukunftsbang

Anxious about the future, atremble about the past.

When Api at last arrived in Suderburg, on Saturday 13 October, I screamed in terror at the gaunt and haggard stranger in his crumpled and grimy clothes. My screams, however, were drowned out by the joy on all sides. He hugged and kissed us all again and again as eventually even I submitted to his embraces. We cried and laughed and talked all at once. Already as he held us close to him, Api felt his thin arms grow stronger. He greeted the Blue Mountain like a long lost friend.

Once we had settled down a bit, the three grown ups spent hours talking about everything that they had gone through. I did not understand what they were saying but felt the joy underlying even the most fearful remembrances. Api sketched in his months in Berlin, which seemed to recede into a strange nightmare even as he was describing them. Nyussi told him about our situation here and the friends she and my mother had made, both with the people of Suderburg and even with the British.

A main topic to which they all came back again and again was the lost past and the loved ones who had been lost with it. In a poem Api wrote later about those first days in Suderburg in October 1945, he used two words that probably characterised their mood. They are *zukunftsbang und vergangenheitdurschauert.* The two typically long German composite adverbs mean 'anxious about the future and atremble about the past'. At that early time neither my grandparents nor my mother had any confidence about what was to become of us. I have a letter my mother wrote to her father-in-law in Vienna in which she described her profound sense of insecurity. A widow at the age of 23 with a small child and without training, as yet, in any profession, her future loomed in menacing uncertainty. The war was over, but they were hungry and cold and had only a tiny place for the four of us. They tried to survive hour by hour worrying about how to provide the next meal and warmth for the two rooms. Thinking about the past was an escape from those anxieties, but it also brought with it a misery of the heart.

Api did not remain long in this state of inactive anxiousness. Now that he was free and united with his family, nothing could hold him back. As he had so often pictured it in his imagination when he was alone in Berlin, he was energised by the reunion and the need to become the provider once again. His path to that was clear: he had to build a practice once more. He would have to work out of the larger of the two cottage rooms we had been given. It was no more than 10sq ft and we ate there and my mother slept in it at night, but Api had learnt in his Begastrasse sub-let how to deal with such constraints. The few instruments he had brought would have to do for now. As soon as he had scraped together a little money he would replenish them. It felt like starting life all over again, which, at the age of 58, was not an easy thing to do. But Api threw himself into the task with energy and even joy, feeling Nyussi's strength at his side.

Before he could start, however, Api had to fight his way through a paper jungle. Documents were required for everything he wanted to undertake. The German bureaucracy was bad enough, but now there was an additional layer of paperwork from the occupiers. He needed a work pass from the employment office and a permit to practise from the Health Bureau. In addition to an identity card from the British zone, he had to obtain a special inter-zone passport allowing him to travel between occupation zones. Even I, a child of only 3, needed a British identification card. I found that small piece of brown cardboard among the papers in my mother's box, together with Api's work pass and inter-zone passport.

Api did not limit himself to waiting for patients to come to his 'surgery'. He made house calls right away. This was important since several villages were spread out in a radius of about 15 miles and almost no one had a car. Patients simply were unable to reach a doctor. The local pastor, Herr Franke, loaned Api an old and rather rickety bicycle which helped Api to get around. He soon was cycling all over the area which, fortunately, was rather flat, although the sandy paths and rough cobblestone roads made it difficult to keep the bike upright. Luckily the winter of 1945 was mild.

Since we were refugees and had almost nothing it was necessary to file applications for every personal and household item. Special tickets were needed for clothing and we were grateful for any used clothing provided by someone's charity. Food, above all, was scarce. The bakers had no flour to make bread, the electricity service was often interrupted and fat was almost impossible to find. We made good use of the thick stand of nettles in the ditch outside our door, although the watery nettle soup, made without fat or flavour, which my mother prepared on our electric burner, was neither tasty nor satisfying. At least it was warm.

I have to smile at this since now, at a time of plenty when just about any delicacy is within my reach, I go hunting for nettles because I have learned how nutritious they are! When we travel to Vienna we seek out a cream-laced bowl of nettle soup at one of our favourite restaurants in the beautiful square of the Grosse Markt. Back then, however, our nettle soup was nothing like this creamy, beautifully pale green concoction. If we were lucky our soup was enhanced with a donation from Nyussi's relations, the Steinkes. When we visited them, farmer Heinrich Steinke's sister Doris often slipped us a piece of sausage, bacon or *Speck*.

In addition to his medical work, Api had an endless series of unaccustomed survival chores, which he undertook with childish glee, perhaps remembering his boyhood in Marienwerder. On weekends we went foraging in the forests for firewood. Occasionally we were lucky to be given some logs from a farmer or a patient and then Api had to split the wood and store it in as dry a place as he could find. Without a shed, that was no easy task in the damp climate. Peat was also welcome when we could get it. Peat burned hot, and for a short while our room was cosy, but it did not burn as cleanly as wood nor did it last as long.

Api's practice grew, but as the months passed he saw that the prospects in Suderburg were limited. It was too small to offer opportunities for seeing more complicated cases or doing surgeries. In order to have more scope for his skills, Api contacted the nearest hospital. This was the Hamburgische Krankenhaus, Hamburg Hospital, in the town of Bevensen less than 20 miles away. When Api went there in the winter of 1946, he was made welcome right away. The hospital needed an eye surgeon and they were pleased to take on a man of Api's reputation. Walking around, Api saw that the hospital consisted of a collection of wood and brick barracks connected by sandy paths in the pine woods outside Bevensen. Yet he found that it was better equipped than anything he had dealt with recently in Berlin. It was, after all, the main hospital of the city of Hamburg. After the bombing of Hamburg in 1943, which had burnt down much of the city in a fierce firestorm, the hospital had been hastily transferred to the safety of the small town where it had had almost three years to establish itself. Becoming part of the team at the Hamburgische Krankenhaus was a stroke of good fortune, which was to help Api for the remainder of his life. He went there from Suderburg at least once a week, often going by bike to save the cost of a train ticket.

Although Api's practice was getting better, we still had little to live on. We shared this fate, of course, not only with almost all refugees, but with most Europeans in that immediate post-war time. Api was thrown back to his earliest years when he had to *knausern*, be stingy, with everything. Every envelope he received was carefully turned over and stuck together inside out so that it could be used again. He urged us to unravel sweaters that had become too small and use the yarn to make something new. Whenever possible we saved on wood for the little iron stove that heated our rooms, since wood was very hard to obtain and even the fallen timber in the surrounding forests was much picked over by the hundreds of other refugees in the neighbourhood. Above all, every piece of fat was used and shared punctiliously, although Api always saw to it, and everyone agreed, that I got more than my share.

In Suderburg Api continued to make house calls. As the weather grew milder in the spring of 1946, he often took me along for company on the back seat of the bike. I had long forgotten that initial shock of seeing him, and had come to adore my Api. With my arms wrapped tightly around his waist on the bike, I listened to him as he talked to me about the plants and trees we were passing. He encouraged me to look closely at everything on our way, the buds on a bush or the placid black-and-white Holstein cows in a field. We played the game of finding the shapes of animals in the clouds. He also told me stories and I loved to listen, although I dimly realised that Api's stories had more of a lesson or message than Nyussi's did. A favourite of his was Aesop's fable of the ant and the grasshopper. Its moral of saving for the future fit so nicely into his own disposition. However, I tended to side with the happy grasshopper who chirped away the summer without a care in the world. It was not easy to get excited about the industrious ant who painstakingly prepared for leaner times. When winter came, in Api's version, the ant complacently told the grasshopper who was starving: 'Well, why don't you chirp now?' Api then turned around on his bike to look at me and asked what I thought was the moral of the story. I had no doubt about Api's preference for the saving ant. I still think so, although his diary now tells me that he loved grasshoppers as the friends of his youth.

With Api there, we made even stronger contacts with the Suderburg elite. Nyussi and Api played bridge with a group of local honoraries that included the mayor whose name I have forgotten, Pastor Franke, the local veterinarian Dr Lorscheid, and Wilhelm and Aline Westermann who lived in *Waidmann's Ruh*, Forester's Rest. It was Suderburg's mansion, situated on the outskirts of the village about 2km beyond our cottage and separated from the road by a park. Aline was the sister of a mining director, now deceased, who had retired there. For me the big place was always surrounded by mystery because the grown ups often talked in whispers about the 'tragedy'. I later found out that some years earlier their young grandchild had fallen into the well and drowned.

Forester's Rest was the favourite spot for bridge games. Afterwards the hostess spread the table with food of a kind we had not tasted in many months, even years. My grandparents stuffed themselves with pork roast, or *Torten*, with whipped cream. On the way home their stomachs, not used to such richness, felt painfully full. Their hosts made sure they had something extra to take back with them as well.

The Christmas of 1945 was nonetheless our poorest ever, but we were so happy to have Api with us that the deprivations became less onerous. He made an Advent wreath out of fir boughs he and I had picked in the woods. He had also saved silver paper, which he now cut into thin strips. His home-made tinsel glittered on the Advent wreath as brightly as the real stuff. We did not have candles for each of the four Advent Sundays, but only one in the centre which burned brightly for all the four weeks. The wreath also served as our Christmas tree that year. The medieval Suderburg church had a big tree with the required twelve candles for the twelve days of Christmas, and we could all enjoy its warm beauty on Sundays. Nyussi did not have a piano nor Api a violin, but we sang Christmas carols together. I chimed in lustily, though out of tune. That year Api did not write a Christmas poem.

48

Return to Blue Mountain

Today we have a joyous celebration on our heath
To which I came when I was very small.

On our trip in the winter of 2008 Mike and I also visited Suderburg in search of Farmer Ohlde's cottage. My son Benedict joined us for this leg of the trip for he wanted to see the places he had heard so much about when he was growing up. It felt good to have them with me, especially since both supported my project and had helped me with it.

I was thrilled as soon as I saw the yellow street sign by the side of the road that announced Suderburg and Mike took a picture of me in front of it. Just seeing the name there made all my thoughts about the place more real. We found the village much as I remembered it, although it had grown on the outskirts. The old church looked more prosperous than in 1945. Its red brick had been beautifully restored and the windows freshly painted white. The rough grey stone tower still looked incongruous but strong, meant to last hundreds more years. The old oaks were there, too, surrounding the church. Even the weather on this day in early January was just what I remembered, chilly and damp, with a slight fog hovering above the meadows.

The most exciting part was still ahead: farmer Ohlde's cottage. I did not remember the streets of Suderburg, but I knew that when we found the cemetery we would be there. Sure enough, we saw the cemetery with its oak trees and the sandy path curving up around it to the village of Holxen where the Steinkes had lived. Across the path we found a richly green and thick stand of nettles. We looked across meadowland to the Blue Mountain; it was much less of a mountain than I had remembered and neither was it blue. We just saw a slight wooded rise in the distance, but still the very words *Blauer Berg* gave me a sense of protection and belonging. I greeted Api's old friend as no doubt he would have done. Farmer Ohlde's small cottage, however, was gone. In its stead and a little further up the Holxen road someone had built a two-storey timbered house. Its red brick and dark timbers looked prosperous and fitted in perfectly with the style of the older homes and farms in this part of northern Germany.

When we drove on to Holxen, we found a picturesque village of half-timbered farmhouses, many of them still with thatched roofs. It was very quiet and no one was about to ask for directions. However, I soon recognised the large old farmhouse of the Steinkes, its cobbled yard bounded on one side by the house and on the other by a big barn. Walking into the farmyard, to the left I saw the steps leading up to what I was sure was the kitchen. It was the way we had always entered. We climbed the steps and knocked hesitantly. After some time we heard slow footsteps approaching and then the door was opened by an elderly woman. I identified myself with a smile and after a moment's hesitation the woman's face lit up. She reached out to hold 'little Gaby' in her arms. She was, I knew, Wilma Förster, the Steinkes' daughter. Well into her eighties, she still was a handsome elderly woman with bright blue eyes, white hair and rosy cheeks. Wilma asked us to come in. Inside, not much had changed either. We still entered the place by the huge kitchen which looked out over moist green meadows. It was sparingly furnished as of old with a large table in the centre and a stove and sink along one wall. A smell of yeast and freshly baked bread or cake pervaded and warmed the large and otherwise rather chilly room. Wilma led the way to the parlour. We passed a smaller room which was dominated by a huge television screen, but otherwise the dark heavy furniture was that of her parents, and perhaps their parents before that.

Wilma invited us to have coffee and *Butterkuchen*, literally butter cake, which I have always loved. That must have been the inviting smell we noticed in her kitchen. *Butterkuchen* is a specialty of the area, made of yeast dough with butter and sugar spread on top. It has to be freshly baked, otherwise it tastes dry and dull, and this one was still warm from the oven. As Mike, Benedict and I were biting into the crusty butter-and-sugar layer of the cake and tasting the soft fluffy inside, I enjoyed listening to Wilma's precise northern German accent, which I had not heard in years. Mike and Benedict, used to my high German, found hers impossible to understand.

Wilma and I started talking almost at once about how I had recited Api's poem at her wedding in 1953 and she brought out an old family album, which showed pictures of me and Api and Nyussi sitting with many other guests in the great hall where the celebration had taken place. I remember that when Api told me that it was time to go on stage I was scared of the large audience. He reassured me that we had practised the poem many times and I would do a fine job. As I walked to the podium, I had the presence of mind to ask the band to play a *Tusch*, a loud sound with cymbals and drums which demands quiet. When silence had fallen and I stood alone on stage in my fancy light-blue dress with ruffles at the knee, I panicked. I started to recite but soon got stuck and Api had to help out from the hall. I must have got through it all for Wilma said that while she did not remember the exact words of the poem, she will never forget the sentiments, not only the good wishes of which it spoke but also the deep sense of gratitude for all the help her family had given the refugees of 1945. I still have the poem, which is conceived from the point of view of myself as 10-year-old girl. It begins with:

> *Today we have a joyous celebration on our heath*
> *To which I came when I was very small.*

Then it goes on to talk about my happy memories of the Steinkes' farm, although I am afraid that in my translation I am unable to recreate the rhyme, in this case following the pattern of abab:

> *When there was loneliness and need in Suderburg*
> *House Steinke always offered open hearts and hands.*

It was only after this expression of thanks that the verses turn to the good wishes for the young couple.

Wilma told me that every time I visited with my grandparents in those days, I soon crawled under the big dining room table with the fringed tablecloth. I did not remember that but assumed that I was continuing my favourite game of playing beaver burrow. I do remember the Steinkes waving us goodbye from the stoop by the kitchen, and one of them handing Nyussi a little parcel of sausage or *Speck*. The women waved their handkerchiefs as long as they could see us. On the walk back to Suderburg we talked of their friendship and what we would do with the treasure they had given us.

Wilma also gave me information on the relatives who had left Holxen in the nineteenth century from whom Nyussi is descended. Luise Hinrichs, Nyussi's grandmother on her father's side, came from a prosperous farm in Holxen, and Nyussi's grandfather August Döhrmann was from the neighbouring village of Hösseringen. He was a *Wiesenbau* engineer, literally a meadow-building engineer, who had studied in the only such school in Germany which happened to be in Suderburg. *Wiesenbau*, which essentially is drainage of meadowlands, is important in that ever-waterlogged area, and the Suderburg school enjoyed an international reputation. After graduation, August emigrated to serve in Turkey under the sultan. His job there was the reverse of what was needed back home. He had to design and build an irrigation system. At some point he came back home to get married. Eventually he left the sultan's employment and settled in Hungary to oversee a horse farm. He must have kept rather close contact with his home, for when his first son Heinrich, Nyussi's father, was born, he sent his wife back to give birth in Hannover, the largest city of his district. Luise's sister had remained in Holxen and married a man by the name of Steinke who owned the largest farm in the village, the place where we now were sitting. They were Wilma's grandparents.

At the end of our visit with Wilma, when we had finished most of the *Butterkuchen* and exhausted our shared memories, Wilma turned to the present. She told us sad but typical stories of a dying village. All the young people were leaving, stores had closed, her old friends were sick or dead and she saw little future for her once prosperous home.

On our way back from Wilma Förster-Steinke we drove by Forester's Rest, having got instructions from Wilma on how to get there. The place looked abandoned and much smaller than I remembered it. The park in front of the house was overgrown with weeds and the fence broken. We had come across another abyss between then and now.

49

Theodor

I have so many loving memories to go home with
which I will cherish always.

The Steinke family was our major support in 1945, but our social
status also helped to make life more bearable. Even before Api had
joined us, Nyussi and my mother, who spoke fluent English, had
made friends with Dave, a British airman. Dave had first come to
our cottage with another airman at the start of the occupation. They held
their rifles at the ready as they were engaged in a house-to-house search of
the village. Nyussi had literally disarmed them when, with a wave of her
hand, she asked them in her broken English: 'Please put that down, it makes
me nervous.' They both laughed and our friendship with Dave began from
that moment. That was even before the order not to fraternise with the
German population had been rescinded, and despite the Ohldes' vociferous
disapproval of our connection with a member of the occupying forces. With
his brown curly hair and always cheerful attitude, Dave reminded Nyussi
of her dead son, and no doubt the young man was glad for a little motherly
nurturing in this foreign country whose language he did not speak. In
fact, Dave soon called Nyussi 'mother' and Api 'father'. Considering that
just weeks before we had been enemies, it is testimony to the human spirit
how quickly individuals can bridge that abyss created by war. It may well

be that this friendship was accelerated because Dave soon began courting my mother.

I remember Dave as a cheerful and boisterous presence in our cottage. Whenever I saw him walk towards us in his airman's blue-grey serge tunic, I ran out to meet him. He twirled me in the air and then we walked into the cottage hand in hand. His laughter filled the small room. Dave exuded health and good spirits, which stood in stark contrast to us hollow-eyed, grey and skinny creatures. And he never came empty-handed. After an affectionate welcome, he pulled a can of meat or a bar of chocolate from his pockets. Most importantly, however, he brought love and acceptance.

A note he wrote to Nyussi when she was in the hospital shows the extent of his love for our family. I copy it in full, and only wish I could thank Dave. I will, however, do what Api suggested in relation to Fräulein Herzog: since I cannot thank him personally, I do so in my heart. Dave wrote:

> I am very happy to have your extremely nice letter from Father and I thank you so much for all you have done and said. – As your son I will remain and my thoughts are with you now and ever. Margit and Father will surely tell you all about my deepest feelings for this dear family. I have so many loving memories to go home with which I will cherish always. Get better soon, Mother Dear. I go, but will return again for certain.
> All my love,
> Dave.

I wonder whether Api and Nyussi were reminded with a pang of pain of Dieter's letter which he ended with 'dead certain'. Dave and Dieter must have been just about the same age.

When Dave returned from a leave in London, he had a special gift for me. I looked at the parcel with great excitement. Gifts were a rarity for me. When I unwrapped it I found a soft, light-blue teddy bear with shiny brown eyes. It instantly became my favourite toy. I don't know whether I loved Theodor because he was my only new toy, or because Dave had given it to me, or because he looked different from German teddies and had come from so far away. Before him I had only one doll, called Henrietta. She was a lanky cloth doll with a painted face for whom Nyussi had made a dress from a skirt I had outgrown. I do not remember why I called her Henrietta, which does not sound like a name for a doll I would have liked, and I am not sure that I ever did like her. She always seemed to be in trouble for I tended to blame Henrietta for anything I had done wrong. At any rate, after Theodor I never looked at Henrietta again and never wanted another doll at all. Theodor was it, as far as I was concerned. I still treasure Theodor today, although he has lost all his hair and sawdust is coming out behind the black stitching of his nose. Now that Api is not there any longer, he cannot fix the one eye Theodor has lost either. But still Theodor has a place of honour on my wardrobe.

After Dave was reassigned some time in 1947, we all missed him very much. Nyussi in particular missed 'our faithful son', as she called him in English. That Christmas we received a beautiful big parcel from him, which contained such precious items as coffee, cocoa and soap. Sadly, all my efforts with the RAF to find out more about Dave have failed since I do not even have his last name. I made many enquiries and posted an announcement in the RAF magazine, but with no result. I would have loved to contact him or, if he is no longer living, his relatives to thank them for all he did and tell him how much it has meant to me and my family.

50

Keep Your Ears Stiff

Shut up and keep serving.

Our food supply improved in the spring and summer of 1946. The Ohldes allowed us to use a corner of their vegetable patch. As we prepared the beds with seeds the Steinkes had given us of peas, carrots and lettuce, the Ohldes looked on suspiciously to see whether these city folks were able to make anything grow. We did, and enjoyed the results for much of the summer and autumn.

My mother earned a little extra money for the family by picking potato beetles off the potato plants for the small farmers of the area. I helped her, and we went side by side down the slightly raised aisles of potato plants. I admired the iridescent beetles which crawled about everywhere on the leaves. Their little black legs stood out in sharp contrast to their shiny and many-coloured bodies. We picked hundreds of them in a day. When the beetle-picking season was over we gathered wild blueberries in the woods. They were small but so much tastier than the cultivated variety. When it was warm enough, Api put a bowl of milk on a windowsill to get sour. For some reason, he always was in charge of the sour milk. When the milk had turned thick and creamy, we ladled it atop the blueberries. It was a wonderful meal and a special treat. The rest of the berries we sold, going from door to door. In the autumn Api and I also went hunting in the woods for lingonberries.

Since I was small, it was easier for me to spot the red berries low to the ground under their shiny green leaves. We did not have much sugar with which to cook them, but I loved their tart flavour and beautiful colour.

The north German summer did not last long and soon the weather turned wet and chilly again. Unlike the previous winter, that of 1946/47 was the harshest anyone could remember. Like everyone else around us, we were hungry and cold. No one had enough heating or food during that grim winter. The progress with Api's practice had also levelled off. Most people were too poor to afford eye treatment. Worn out by years of malnutrition, it seemed to Api that he would never be able to provide adequately for us. After a nettle or potato soup and perhaps a cup of *Muckefuck*, we all crawled into our beds early to try to stay warm. My place still was in the middle between Api and Nyussi in the smaller of the two rooms, and they helped to keep me warm. It was a time, as Api later reflected, of boundless hopelessness, but for me there were also happy moments. Calling to Nyussi, 'let's be cosy', we cuddled up together. If I was lucky she had an apple which she put on the stove to bake. While the aroma drifted through the little room, Nyussi told me fairy tales. When the apple was soft and warm, she divided it and we played dominoes while we savoured the treat. Api had taught me the game early on for he saw it as another way to teach me about numbers, and he was proud at how quickly I picked it up.

The worst part of that winter was Nyussi's illness. She had developed rheumatoid arthritis which, coupled with poor nutrition and years of stress, caused a series of infections that affected many organs. She was always in pain and had a low-grade fever for weeks, and yet whenever she could manage at all she distracted herself from her pain with her favourite pastime: reading. She had borrowed the first volume of Carl J. Burckhardt's *Richelieu* as well as Leopold von Ranke's classic *Roman Popes in the Last Four Centuries*. At one point she was delighted when she caught the author out with a wrong date. Eventually she had to be hospitalised in the Hamburgische Krankenhaus in Bevensen, where she stayed for an entire year. For a time we feared for her life. We missed her good spirits and support. Without her the cottage was bleak.

Strangely, the hospital decided to take out all Nyussi's teeth, which were seen as the heart of the infection. Api did not understand why that had to be done, but the specialist who treated Nyussi insisted on it. Until the wounds in her gums had healed, she was without any teeth and after that she suffered through a series of ill-fitting prostheses. As a result, she could eat only soups, porridge and mashed foods, and lost even more weight.

We visited her often in the hospital to make her feel better, but it was Nyussi who tried to keep our spirits up rather than the other way around. She did not complain about her pain. At most she said jokingly about her position: 'How was it in my *au devant* fatherland: "*Maul halten and weiter dienen.*"' Her former, *au devant* fatherland – a French phrase – was the Austro-Hungarian Empire in which she had grown up. What she learnt derives from military parlance and translates to 'shut up and keep serving'. While the grown ups talked by Nyussi's bedside, I remember hop-scotching around the wooded paths that wound between the barracks, and the nurses handing me the delicacy, which I had not known before, of crisp bread with a little pat of butter. I kept coming back for more. Like potatoes with salt, it remains one of my favourite treats.

When we could not visit Nyussi, we wrote to her. At first it had to be postcards only since nothing else was allowed by the censor. Nyussi marvelled at the odd cards she received almost every day. On the top we had to note in what language or, in our case, languages we had written them. Mail from Germany and Austria was censored for years after the war. Api wrote in German in the same tiny script with which he had filled his diary. My mother tended to use Hungarian in her larger, forceful and slanted hand, and Dave always added a few tender words in English to 'Mother', scribbled in his spidery scrawl. I wonder whether these trilingual postcards attracted the censor's attention.

On Christmas Eve 1946 I recited Api's poem of the year, which indicates that he saw some hope, without which he could not go on. I doubt I understood much of it as I voiced the lines I had learnt by heart, but it is Api's first Christmas poem in my possession and the first one I recited at the age of 4. The poem ends with:

> *They* [angels] *bring after bitterest blows of fate*
> *once again light for us in the darkness*
> *Humility, patience, and contentment!*
> *Listen and believe – that is Christmas blessing.*

Again, in trying to capture the meaning of the poem, my translation loses the rhyme and also some of the meter. This time Api had written the poem in the form of abba and in an elegiac meter.

When the long and cold winter of 1946/47 at last came to an end, Api's spirits picked up. Despite the hardships and Nyussi's continued illness, spring invariably brought new hope, refreshing him in body and soul. As the elders and willows along the Hardau creek began to grow green, as the earthy smell of the fields drifted over to our cottage and the woods of the Blue Mountain reawakened, he wrote that 'despite everything the world is immeasurably beautiful'. With trust in God and hard work he felt there was yet hope for a more secure future. '*Ohren steif halten*', the German version of a stiff upper lip, was his motto, which literally translates to 'keep your ears stiff'. It was one of Api's favourite sayings. What always followed immediately was 'and thank the Lord with all our hearts for what He still has left us and in many respects already given us again'. His life had been reduced to terror and anxiety for so long that he felt exhilarated by the return to a fuller existence where he could once again take care of his family.

51

Kindertransport

I would have liked best to send you my old mother's
heart along with this letter. Even the dear censor may
have let it through.

In the spring of 1947 my mother left for Vienna. Except for lowly jobs
like picking potato beetles, Suderburg had no opportunities for her
whatsoever. Vienna, although derelict and under Allied occupation,
had more to offer her. Brought up in Berlin, she missed the big city
and her parents-in-law urged her to move and would be there to help her
get ēstablished. My Viennese grandfather, a former general, pulled some
strings from his pre-war army days and managed to get her an apartment
in the Arsenal, a huge complex in the south-east of Vienna near the South
railway station. It was built in 1848 and served as a barracks and armoury
during the First World War. Each building, or *Projekt* as it was called, looked
like a modern-day castle built of red brick with sandstone decorations and
broad stone stairways and turrets. Much of the Arsenal had been damaged
during the war, but it was gradually being rebuilt. When she first lived
there, in *Projekt XIV*, my mother had to walk through a field of rubble to
get to her building. This was particularly scary at night, especially since
the occupation forces were still around. But her apartment was on the top
floor from where she could just catch a glimpse of St Stephen's Cathedral in

the centre of Vienna. With her language skills – she was fluent in French, English and Hungarian – she soon found work: first as secretary, then as translator of business correspondence at the 'Abadie', a factory that made cigarette paper.

The spring of 1947 brought a pleasant even if short-lived surprise for Api in Suderburg. For almost a year he had made applications for a new bike to use for his visits to patients. At last, after pages and pages of documents, he was granted special permission to obtain a new bike by no less than the President of Lower Saxony. He had to go to Lüneburg, the district centre, to pick it up. The bike was a local brand he had never heard of called Heidemann, but it served him well and was the envy of the neighbours. So much so, in fact, that it was stolen a few months later.

We all missed my mother but especially Nyussi, who was still confined to her hospital room. To cheer up her daughter in Vienna she wrote letters full of funny scenes and word plays, of courage and confidence, and they all testified that her main concern was her daughter's welfare. My mother obviously cherished those letters for she stowed them away in her lockbox, so that now I am able to hear Nyussi's voice over the decades. When my mother had trouble at her first job, Nyussi encouraged her not to fall victim to existential *Angst* but to hold her head high and have faith in the future, a belief which, she insisted, was not just a sign of her Hungarian reckless spirit. She added, 'In confidence, in this way I have also been able to help your dear father when he was down emotionally. Now he sits again firm in the saddle.' Reflecting on the past years, she wrote: 'It is bad luck that we lost everything. So now we just have to start anew. We will make it somehow.'

Api's Christmas poem of 1947 reflects our family's ambivalent mood. It tells of anxiety and hardship before it ends with the Christmas message of peace and hope. The opening lines say:

> *Dark lies Christmas over cold and wintry heath*
> *Oh, so great are human woes*
> *And so many a sad tear flows*
> *Even today when God sent the highest joy.*

Once my mother was established, she sent for me. The only way I could get to Vienna was in a *Kindertransport*, a children's transport. The

Rückführungsschein, the document which allowed me to travel to her, indicated that the transport would be free of vermin and infectious diseases but that I needed provisions for at least two days. We were travelling in a goods train. Our wagon was crowded with kids between, I think, the ages of 5 and 15. I certainly remember that I was one of the youngest. The wagon floor was covered in a thick layer of straw and there were no seats. However, we had a nurse or a teacher who played games with us. The train made slow progress with many delays. Whenever we came to a long stop on the open tracks or pulled on to a side rail we were allowed out to run about and play under the supervision of the teacher.

My mother picked me up at the Western station in Vienna and I was awestruck by its huge glass dome. Then we had a wonderful weekend together. My mother took me to the Cobenzl, Vienna's *Hausberg*, its local mountain from where we could look out over Vienna. I had never seen such a big city: so many buildings, red-roofed houses, church spires, factories and such a big river snaking through it. Sitting on a grassy meadow looking out on this marvel, she opened a pointed brown paper bag, which had little rough beige-coloured shapes inside. She cracked one open and gave it to me to eat. It was my first peanut, but try as I might I could not open one for myself.

After the weekend my mother had to board me since she was working all day. Again with my paternal grandfather's aid, she had found a place for me at the prestigious convent school run by Ursuline nuns, the very school where my great-grandmother had been educated. It was located in a small and dark Renaissance building on the Genzgasse in Vienna's eighteenth district. The nuns offered an excellent but stern education. In first grade I learnt to read and write fluently, as well as to knit and crochet. The convent rules were very strict, however. You were not allowed to talk in the corridors, and had to fold your clothes and make your bed in a very precise manner. We slept in a large hall on the second floor of the two-storey building. The hall had a low ceiling and my bed, ignominiously, was the only one with a rail around it because I was small and much younger than the others. The nuns made an austere and frightening impression on me as they walked about in their heavy black serge habits, which fell in folds to their feet. Their heads were encased in a white wimple which left only their eyes, mouth and nose visible. When I was afraid of the dark, a nun, her face framed by the stiff white linen with the starched white yoke around her neck sticking out sharply at me, said in a stern voice: 'It is only your own bad deeds which make you afraid.' The convent re-baptised me, now already 6 years old, into the Catholic faith and later I was also confirmed in the Catholic tradition, wearing a fancy white lace dress and holding a large decorated candle.

In the spring of 1948 Nyussi was finally released from the Bevensen hospital. She still was in pain and her arthritis had deformed her hands and feet, but at least she was home. Api was ecstatic to have her back. The living and work space in the Suderburg cottage was tiny, but Nyussi was determined to make it as comfortable as she could. My grandparents could once more enjoy their afternoon coffees together, even if it was only *Muckefuck*. On the rare occasions when Nyussi was allowed to use Frau Ohlde's stove, she baked a *Streussel* cake or a *kolacz*, the Hungarian sweet white bread. When they sat together of an evening, and especially if Api had managed to scare up a cigar, they were grateful for the life they had. The rain and wind might beat at their little window, but they were cosy inside. This was true especially after Nyussi, believing that Api was overdoing his *knausern* by saving too much wood, had taken over as 'heat director', as she called it. They sat together by the warm stove, talked about the past and made plans for what they now confidently felt would be a better future.

The only people missing from their contentment were me and my mother in Vienna. The letters they wrote all testify how much they missed me in particular. Every one of them has repeated references to 'our most beloved little Gaby', 'our sweetest sunshine', 'whom we remember at every step and who again and again makes our old hearts ring in painful longing'. In one letter of March 1949 Api exclaimed, 'O little Gaby, little Gaby if only you could have been there with us' when they visited a fair. Or he talked about the bike rides we could take and in autumn, when the acorns were particularly big, about the acorn pipes we could cut. He also wrote letters to me full of love and admonishments to do well in school.

Nyussi continued the frequent correspondence with her only surviving child that she had begun in the hospital. It had been more than a year since my mother had left and Nyussi so wanted to see her. In the summer of 1948 she begged my mother to visit. She hoped to entice her by saying that we would all take a holiday together at the North Sea: 'After your dog's life, a few weeks of a seal's life [in German seal is 'sea dog'] will do you much good.' But my mother could not get away. Nyussi wrote in response to that disappointing news: 'I am with you so much in my thoughts that I shouldn't be surprised if you noticed my astral body crouching in a corner of your sofa.' Responding to a despondent letter from my mother, Nyussi tried to inspire courage and support, and ended with: 'I hope I was able to write as I feel. I would have liked best to send you my old mother's heart along with this letter. Even the dear censor may have let it through.'

With Nyussi back home and spring well on the way, Api, always inclined to sentimental attachments, waxed quite emotional about life in their new home on the heath. In May 1948 he wrote to my mother in Vienna:

> The heather which lies immediately outside our window and also already in our hearts, is beautiful, and beautiful, too – despite everything – is life which still has left us the community of dearly loved ones and the possibility of grateful remembrance and prayer.

He had even come to love the fog which spread such silence all around:

> The pale silhouettes of the trees seem like an unfinished etching and the fog immediately devours even the lamplight which, so familiar and alluring, seeps out of warm rooms.

After less than two years with the Ursulines, I became seriously ill. It began with diarrhoea and a high fever. I soiled my bed and one of the nuns picked me up in the middle of the night and, in view of all the other students, held me under a cold-water tap to clean me off. It was not a good start, but it got worse. I became delirious and the convent nursery could no longer handle my case. In the hospital I was diagnosed with scarlet fever. They also suspected pneumonia and I was put under quarantine for months. I could see my mother only through a glass wall, and we 'touched' by placing our hands on the same spot on either side of the glass partition. When I was over the worst, I was transferred to the only place where they could find me a bed. It was at Steinhof, on a hill at the edge of the Vienna Woods and it overlooked the city, but Steinhof was a hospital for the mentally ill. When

I got better and could leave my room, I was amused as well as frightened by the strange people I saw walking about.

My grandparents pleaded with my mother to send me back to Suderburg. They felt that they could take care of me better than she was able to as a working mother on her own. Api urged that living with them in a stable home surrounded by love would help 'my beloved little soul' recover faster since 'as is well known both in illness and recovery the mind and the spirit have an extraordinary influence on the functioning of our organism'. He added that with all their infinite love my education would not lack the necessary seriousness either. Eventually my mother agreed that the country air and the care of my grandparents would do me good. I was sent from Vienna in another children's transport. Somehow I got stuck at the station in Hannover, about 62 miles (100km) away. Fortunately, someone sent a telegram to the address I carried around my neck saying that I was at the station mission. Api jumped on a train immediately, reaching Hannover at 3 a.m., but there was no sign of me. After a search of several hours, he found me in a women and children's bunker among a collection of other lost children. It was a happy reunion with my Api, and I clutched him tightly, afraid we would be separated. The sun was just coming up as we boarded the train for the ride back to Suderburg. Sitting on my little wooden suitcase I fell asleep almost immediately, still holding on to him.

I was delighted to be back with Api and Nyussi. Even the Ohldes welcomed me and I was glad to see the familiar farmyard with my old friends, the Ohldes' dog, whose name I have forgotten, and Lotte the sheep. Once again I watched farmer Ohlde go out to tend his bees, dressed all in white with a big net over his head, and although I was no longer starving, I followed him as of old as he fed the pigs. From a letter Nyussi wrote to my mother I learned that I continued to talk to the animals, as I had done before I left. I conversed not only with the dog and the sheep, but with the bees and the chickens and the birds. Today I am pleased to see that my habit of talking to animals goes back to my earliest youth. That day Nyussi reported I had come in telling her that I just talked to a blackbird and he told me that summer would come soon.

52

De-Nazified

Exonerated!

The procedure of releasing Germans from their *Pg* status continued for years after the war. The process was still much the same as it had been set up in 1946. The applicant had to write a detailed letter describing his activities during the Nazi period and he had to provide testimonies from others corroborating or adding to what he had said. A commission looked into each case and classified the applicant according to five categories established by the Allies in Directive 38 on 12 October 1946: Chiefly Responsible, Incriminated, Less Incriminated, Fellow Traveller and Exonerated.

Here is my last discovery about Api's past. Among his papers in my mother's box I found his de-Nazification document, dated 19 May 1949. It said that Api had not been active in the Nazi Party and had continued to treat Jewish patients. As a result he was classified in the lowest of the five categories as *Entlasteter*, which means exonerated or, literally, 'unburdened'. Api no doubt felt that indeed a burden had been lifted when he received that judgement. Exoneration must have been a huge relief after years of feeling persecuted and treated like an inferior person, if not a criminal. It was a huge relief even to me so many years later. Exonerated has a good sound to it, even though I realise that these categories cannot be taken fully at their face value. Ultimately, it is clear that Api did not play any active part in the Nazi regime, other, of course, than having become a member on 1 May 1933. Although I was very happy to have found that document of exoneration, I realised that it would not relieve me of my need to account for our shared Nazi past.

Four days after Api's exoneration, on 23 May 1949, the *Grundgesetz*, literally the Basic Law, came into being and the *Bundesrepublik Deutschland* was born. The preamble states: 'Aware of its responsibility before God and men and inspired by the desire to serve world peace in a unified Europe, the German people, through its constitutional powers, has given itself these basic laws.' Germany clearly wanted to close the chapter of Nazi persecution forever and make a new start committed to respecting and protecting each citizen within the state. The German constitution, which was published on that same day, begins with: 'The dignity of human beings is inviolable. To honour and to protect it is the responsibility of all the power of the state.'

53

A Stable Home

Dr. med Herbert Frese, Ophthalmologist

B y 1949 we felt intolerably cramped in the two rooms of the farmhouse and after four years of housing strangers, the Ohldes understandably wanted us out. Api also needed greater scope for his practice than the village of Suderburg, and the commutes to the hospital in Bevensen had become rather arduous. But, try as he might, he could not find accommodation anywhere in the area. He then travelled to various other towns in search of a good place to settle where he knew that an eye doctor was needed, but he met everywhere with the same problem: no place to live. Apartment space was difficult to get in those years when the bombed-out buildings had not yet been restored. Since their chances did not seem any better anywhere else, my grandparents decided to stay. Bevensen, the town with a good hospital where Api already was known, seemed the best option. Once that decision was made, Api kept filling out one application after another. He wrote to the mayor of Bevensen, to the district Housing Bureau, to the Minister of Reconstruction, and even to the President of Lower Saxony in search of a more permanent place. He wrote letters, filled out myriad questionnaires and was engaged in constant negotiations before he was finally successful in the summer of 1949.

When Api was given his verdict of Exonerated we still lived in the Suderburg cottage, but two months later we finally were able to move to a bigger place. I wonder whether not having had such a de-Nazification document until then had anything to do with Api's difficulties in obtaining a place to live. The new apartment consisted of the ground floor of a house in Bevensen at Eckermannstrasse 9 with the owners, the Obstfelders, living on the top floor. The house was on a quiet residential street halfway between the town and the Ilmenau River. Our front windows looked out on the meadows, which sloped to the river and the pine woods of the *Klaubusch* rising steeply on its other side. Api now had a waiting room and surgery and the Obstfelders allowed him to affix a black-and-white enamel sign saying 'Dr. med Herbert Frese, Ophthalmologist' to the slatted fence outside. We also had a good-sized living room. Although there was not enough space for me to have a room of my own, I liked sleeping in my grandparents' room, where the Hinzpeter painting of the Chiemsee hung over their bed and I had a smaller one by the window. Nyussi was delighted that she finally had her own kitchen again. Almost best of all, the apartment came with a tiny Linden arbour in the back which was part of the rental. My grandparents loved to sit there of an afternoon enjoying the tranquil scene among the trees, looking out on the green meadows and reflecting on how fortunate they were to have once again such a nice home.

At this time Helga Friedel joined our household. Nyussi's arthritis continued to worsen and she needed help taking care of the bigger place we now had. She also had been used to having a maid since she was a little girl on her Hungarian estate. Helga was a strong and attractive young woman who had lost both her parents in the war. Her dark blonde hair was cut short, parted at the side and set in curls around her head. Her blue-grey eyes looked straight and fearlessly at the world. She soon became part of the family and stayed with us until Api's death. After that we could not pay her any more and she eventually got married and set up a household of her own. Nyussi corresponded with her until her own death in 1958.

For me, one big event of that year was that I learnt to ride a bike. All we had was an old adult bike and I was so small that my head barely reached above the handle bars. Of course, it was Api who ran alongside my wobbly pedalling, holding on firmly to the saddle. Then he would let go for a few seconds, still running beside me and grabbing the bike when I threatened to topple. Gradually the periods grew longer and soon I was sailing along happily on the cinder paths, up and down Eckermannstrasse or down a small incline to the Ilmenau River. I practised riding without holding on to handle bars and still fell now and then. My knees were permanently crusted with scabs.

At Christmas we discovered a beautiful Bevensen tradition. My grandparents had always attended an afternoon service on Christmas Eve, but this one was special. It was the *Siebenstern* celebration. A *Siebenstern* is a tall seven-sided wooden candlestick, and we soon owned our own. As we entered, the church was completely dark and the service was held without any lights. I could hear the rustle of the large congregation – everyone came to this event – but I could not make out anyone's face. Only at the end of the service did we all light our seven-sided candlesticks and the whitewashed walls of the simple church suddenly shone warmly in the light of hundreds of candles. It was so beautiful, I almost forgot my excitement about the *Bescherung*, the gift-giving to come and the lit tree. On our walk back from the church, first through the little town and then along the dark lane to our house, however, I could think of little else.

It was my first stable home and my grandparents were wonderful, taking care of me with so much love and attention. Despite her worsening arthritis, Nyussi was a lively and spirited grandmother and we laughed a lot together. I still see her coming back from the little town, walking slowly on the sandy path that led from town to Eckermannstrasse, holding a netted shopping bag. She had trouble carrying groceries in her arthritic hands but she never forgot to add something special for me: a caramel, a piece of liquorice or a banana.

Nyussi was a wonderful storyteller. I loved to listen to her slightly accented German as she talked to me about her Hungarian childhood. I especially remember stories about her eccentric uncle Dionysius Farago, whom everyone called Dinybasci. He was a lifelong bachelor who lived with his valet in one wing of their villa in Nagykörös, where he and his sister, Nyussi's mother, owned an estate. Educated as a lawyer, he did not practise a day in his life except to oversee his estate. Although he had lost a good deal of his investments in war bonds, enough was left to afford him a comfortable and easy-going life, which he allowed nothing to upset. Nyussi told me that when one evening he was handed a telegram at the dinner table, he simply laid it aside and continued his meal. Finally, his sister, Nyussi's mother, could not hold back any longer: 'Dinybasci, do open that telegram. It must be urgent.' Uncle Dinybasci looked at her over the glass of Tokay wine he had just raised to his lips and answered, 'Urgent, yes, but for the one who sent it.' He was a big man with a voracious appetite. 'A duck,' he liked to say, 'is an inconvenient bird: one is not enough for one person and two are too much.' Dinybasci loved his horse-drawn carriages and made sure that the horses were matched in size and colour. When she visited, he would take Nyussi and later also my mother and uncle on rides into the vineyards for a picnic or into town for a shopping spree. My mother particularly liked to visit the shoemaker who made her ankle boots of the softest leather that were the envy of her friends in Berlin. I have a picture of Dinybasci's summer carriage. It has small wooden wheels in front and larger ones in the back, and an elegantly curved body with a turned-down hood. Nyussi is reclining in the back seat, her long legs crossed at the knee. She is wearing a dark beret and smiles at the camera. Her uncle is sitting at a small table next to the carriage, probably enjoying a snack. He has his back toward Nyussi but is looking around at her, his face turned away from the camera. He is wearing a bowler hat and frock coat and looks small and rotund. They must be in one of their vineyards for in the background are two workmen standing by three large wooden wine barrels and a one-storey white service building. The whole area is shaded by what look like fig and walnut trees.

Whenever Nyussi talked of her home town Nagykörös she always mentioned the sunny warmth of the broad streets and the vineyards, where apricots, peaches and almonds grew between the vines. It sounded exotic to me for the colder north-German climate produced mainly apples, pears, cherries and currants; even the strawberries had a hard time ripening. Today I wish, however, that Nyussi had told me more about her childhood, or rather that I had asked her more questions about that time. But I preferred the fairy tales she always told me at bedtime. My favourite was *Puss in Boots*, which she had to repeat over and over again although I already knew it by heart.

I basked in all the care and attention and enjoyed the freedom of the small town where I could cycle everywhere on my own. I loved the meadows in front of our house, full of flowers in spring when I brought home fistfuls of anemones and primroses. In summer I hunted for *Sauerampfer*, stacking its bitter but juicy leaves so that I could bite through many layers at once. I built forts in the tall grass near the river and in winter sledded on the steep hill in the woods across the way. There were no pressures on me as yet. Elementary school was easy for me. Thanks to the nuns' superior education, I was well ahead of my class in all subjects, even though I was too sloppy to master the *Sütterlin* script. Looking back now, and even then, it seemed like an idyllic time; after all that had happened, a fairy-tale life.

54

Api and Me

Just as the Lord's all encompassing love
Returns to us each Christmas day …

As I was to discover all too soon, Api was the centre of that fairy tale. He was both father and grandfather to me, spoiling me with love and laughter but also establishing firm rules and discipline. I wanted to be in his company as much as possible. When my teddy bear Theodor's eyes needed mending, I went to Api's surgery so that Theodor could receive proper treatment. I also liked to watch Api as he practised his own surgery skills using pigs' eyes. He had a standing order for them with the local butcher and we went together to collect them, taking them back to the surgery where Api started to work. When he was done he let me look through a magnifying glass at his operation and I marvelled at the tiny incisions. Api did increasingly more eye surgeries at the Bevensen hospital and wanted to be sure his hand was practised and steady. Every evening before bed he and I played dominoes or a card game for two called 66. Api liked 66 because it forced me, always a scatter brain, to concentrate. If I wanted to compete I had to memorise cards and learn to do quick additions. Every card has a different point value and I had to remember how many points I had taken in my tricks. If the total added up to 66, I shouted out '66' and won.

As much as he played games with me, Api's first priority was my education. He never felt that I got enough homework at the Bevensen grade school. So he gave me additional dictation or maths tasks to do, always with the promise of a game afterwards. Whenever possible he tried to make even play educational, such as in 66, and on our outings he always found something to explain. He talked about the seasons, about the animals we saw, or the history of our town and church. We listened to classical music together and early on Api gave me a recorder to develop my musical ear. After church each Sunday he expected me to give a summary of Superintendent Stünkel's sermon. I am afraid I almost always disappointed him. All this may sound a little too schoolmasterish, but Api managed to make it all enjoyable. I never felt lectured or talked down to. Instead, Api taught me to find interest, enchantment even, in the everyday. When we had to wait at the train station, Api helped me while away the time by asking me to draw what I saw in the waiting room. We then discussed what I had chosen and he ended by admiring my 'little work of art' and suggested that I send it to my mother in Vienna.

The one thing Api hated was vacuity. The only times I saw him angry at me was when I was neither working nor playing, but just doing nothing:

> You don't have to work all the time. Play is good. But do not waste your time and the beautiful day like this. If you do not know what to do with yourself, write something about why there are storms in spring and what good they do. Or read one of the books I gave you.

When I did not like any of his suggestions, he often would start a game with me which I did like, but Api never relented in instructing me not to waste time. In a letter he wrote to Nyussi when she and I were visiting friends he suggested:

> If she does not have anything at all to do in her free time, you may perhaps now and then give her an extensive dictation. You best buy an exercise book without lines so that she also learns to write straight. What is important is to write relatively quickly and clearly, and with the least number of mistakes possible. Perhaps you can bring the book back with you so that I, too, can enjoy the results.

In the autumn I particularly enjoyed our building a kite together in the cellar. Api selected two strips of bare wood, testing them for flexibility. He nailed them together into a cross and carefully checked the balance. It had to be exactly right, otherwise the kite would not fly. Next came the delicate task of stretching paper across the surface. We painted big black eyes and red ears on the paper: a dragon's face, since the German word for kite is *Drachen*, or dragon. I had to be careful not to pierce the stretched paper in any spot. It was my job also to make the dragon's tail by folding and tying pieces of newspaper to a string like a series of bow ties. When it was done, we looked at our handiwork and were very pleased. Although by then it usually was too late to fly the kite so we just took it upstairs to show to Nyussi.

I remember one blustery autumn afternoon when we were out in the meadows in front of the house with our newest kite. Api was running as fast as he could to get the kite started. Then, for a moment, he looked up as a patient waved to him from the street. Before he could shout a 'hello', I saw him disappear. I ran to the spot where I had last seen him. Api had fallen into one of the many drainage ditches that dissected the meadow. He sat up in the muddy ditch and I saw him bent over with laughter. He still held on to the kite string and the wind had taken the kite high up into the sky. I tried to hold the string, but the pull was too strong. So, wet as he was, Api anchored our kite deep in the soft soil of the meadow and we watched it bouncing and surging high above us in the air. It looked so small and yet so strong. I could not believe that we had made it ourselves.

In an effort to teach me to make what he considered the right choices, Api often would give me an option: shall we first do our Latin, maths, dictation or whatever homework I needed to finish, or shall we play first? Needless to say I invariably and without hesitation picked the latter. He always honoured my choice but today I can imagine how he must have hoped that just once I would put work before play. When Api took me to Hamburg to show me the beautiful city with its two lakes and great harbour, he again offered me an alternative to round out our day. We could either go to the opera for Verdi's *La Forza del Destino* or we could go to Millöcker's light operetta *The Beggar Student*. Although I knew that Api would much prefer the Verdi, I asked to see the operetta. He must have been disappointed but he never let on and we went to *The Beggar Student*. I may never then have made the choices Api had in mind. However, without realising it, I did absorb most of his gentle teaching, not only his dedication to work but also his enjoyment of play and devotion to nature.

In Bevensen Api revived the family tradition of Sunday outings, and he made each one festive and enjoyable, as well as educational for me. Before we had a car, we went on hikes. A favourite walk took us to Kloster Medingen just outside Bevensen. It was a Cistercian nunnery, founded in 1336. To get there we had to pass a broad alley lined by majestic beeches. On the way Api told me about the nuns who had lived at that place since about 1235:

> The first nuns who lived here had a scary and lonely time. They had no nunnery yet but lived in cottages on the heath, much like the one we had in Suderburg, remember? But Medingen also had a castle with knights. When the nuns got really scared they sought the protection of the knights of Medingen. It took them about 100 years until they finally had their own nunnery. Then life got easier. The nunnery became famous in the area and was part of the six Nunneries of the Heath ... Unfortunately only a brew house has survived from medieval times. Everything else has burnt down over the centuries. Fires were common back then and the old places have been replaced with the newer buildings you now see.

I particularly liked the baroque church because it was round and I had never seen a round church before.

From Medingen we crossed the Ilmenau River at the King's Bridge and followed a small path to the *Nixengrund*, the Mermaid's Hollow. I always hurried through this quiet and eerie spot and, far ahead of Api, climbed to the *Sängershöhe*, the Singers' Hill, above the short but steep Ilmenau shore. The reward for all this exertion was coffee and plenty of *Butterkuchen*.

In 1950, when cars were not yet common, Api bought his first post-war car, a 1948 used grey Opel Olympia. It had done 38,000km and cost 3,000 Marks. The *Grey Donkey* was not as big or as flashy as the Buicks had been, but we all loved it. The car relieved Api of his bike rides to patients and our outings now had a wider range. On Sundays we drove into the Lüneburg Heath, especially to the nearby Göhrde with its sandy paths, birch trees and stunted juniper bushes. Occasionally we saw a shepherd outlined against the sky, standing very still and wearing some long, dark garb. In his hand he held a gnarled crook. It was curved at the top and so long that the curve extended far above the shepherd's head. Api told me that this scene with the shepherd had remained the same for centuries. My attention, however, was focused on the rather small dog that tended the sheep. I was amazed how cleverly he could make the sheep go wherever he wanted.

If Api had not enough time for a longer outing we visited the neighbouring woods, the Riessel and the Lohn, where we looked for mushrooms or gathered pine cones for the fire. Both these woods were locally famous for their tall stands of beech and oak trees. Much like the Grunewald, they, too, had been hunting grounds of the local aristocracy and, therefore, could not be cut down. Api pointed out the stately beauty of the grey-barked beech trees and the delicate green of the larches in spring, making me run my hand across the soft new growth. Walking through even rows of straight, tall stems, Api asked me whether I too felt like I was in a high-arched Gothic cathedral. I wonder now whether he thought of his early poem in which he compared being out in nature to a church service. The poem, with the title 'I Do Not Regret', contains the lines:

> I do not regret a single day that I have swarmed through the hills and valleys of God's beautiful world ... It was neither a church service sitting in a pew nor a day's work in the yoke of duty, but I believe that God also holds school in His creation. I do not regret.

Christmas was Api's special time and he made it special for me. It was he who hunted for the prettiest tree and when he found the one he liked best, cut it down, brought it home and hid it away. On Christmas Eve he decorated it in secret with tinsel, baubles and sweets. None of us was allowed to see the tree until after the Christmas Eve *Siebenstern* service. Back home, Api disappeared into the Christmas room. I heard rustling and motion and listened intently for the tinkling of the little brass bell on the tree, which told us that we could enter. I was the first in the room and was awed by the glow of the twelve candles, the glitter and the presents around the tree.

The Christmas season also was the only time Api was busy in the kitchen, which he otherwise only entered to compliment Nyussi on the cake she had baked or to find out what smelled so good. During the four weeks of Advent he made sure that we had all the ingredients to make marzipan: the almonds, confectioner's sugar and especially the rose water. It was a sign that work was over and the holiday had begun when Api came into the kitchen to make marzipan. He mixed the dough and kneaded it vigorously. Then he fashioned delicate flowers out of the marzipan mixture, using his cast-off surgical instruments to make them as detailed and precise as possible. He also created little marzipan tartlets with carefully fluted edges, which he first baked a golden brown. After they had cooled down he filled them with white icing and then decorated them with sugar ornaments: bells, boughs and stars. We all loved his Christmas marzipan, although Nyussi sometimes got fed up with the mess he made in her kitchen. After the marzipan came the eggnog, or egg liqueur, which Api made after a recipe of his mother's. I, too, was allowed a little glass of the strong creamy concoction with glowed a rich yellow in my glass.

The Christmas poem for 1951 shows how much better things were for Api and all of us. It has no more echoes of terrors overcome and blows of fate, but concentrates on love and faith. The last stanza I recited that year says:

> *Just as the Lord's all encompassing love*
> *Returns to us each Christmas day*
> *So I will pray that from above*
> *Its power remains with us to stay.*

55

Eckermannstrasse 19

A home of our own

The rented floor on Eckermannstrasse 9 was a huge step forward from the one-and-a-half rooms in Suderburg. However, Api's financial situation continued to improve in the time of economic growth, the economic miracle of the 1950s, and the owners of the house had hinted more than once that they would like their ground floor back to themselves. So we were looking for even better accommodation. After many a calculation and discussion with Nyussi, Api decided that we could afford to buy a house of our own. He soon found just the one he wanted. It was at the further end of Eckermannstrasse at No. 19, with the same vista of meadows and woods that we had come to love. Since it was the last house on the street its view was unencumbered on three sides.

When Api showed it to me, saying that this may become our place, I was excited. I loved the house at first sight. It looked so big and solid; its rough stucco painted grey, its steep red-tiled roof and bay windows trimmed in dark wood. The house also had a terraced garden framed by a beech wood hedge and there was a little pond at the bottom. And, even better than the arbour at the Obstfelders, this house had a tiled veranda overlooking the garden. It was open to the sun but sheltered by the house on three sides from the chilly north German winds. In summer, tall blue delphiniums grew right up to the walls. The house even had a drive-in garage into the basement, a very modern amenity in Germany at that time. Other rare advantages were its two and a half bathrooms, one with a large tiled shower room. Bennecke, a local architect, had built the house for himself, but had to sell it before it was completed. So Api was able to purchase it for 32,000 Marks. The garage was unfinished, some windows still had to be installed as well as the upstairs flooring, and we needed a wooden fence around the property. None of this stopped Api for a moment, for I think he was even more excited by the prospect of owning his own home for the first time in his life than I was.

We moved in the summer of 1952. With two separate front entrances, the house was perfect for Api's surgery and for our living. The large living room looked out on the veranda and along the south side of the house stretched a sunny 'winter garden', where Nyussi grew her favourite cyclamens and fuchsias all year round. There also was space for a piano there, although her hands were too crippled to play. I am afraid my childish and not-very-talented attempts to play were, despite regular piano lessons, no substitute. We ate in a cosy wood-panelled den off the kitchen. I spent much of that summer by the pond trying to train the many green frogs that hopped along its edge to jump into bark boats Api and I had made for them. On summer evenings the frogs gave a concert by the pond and later that winter I skated there.

Both my grandparents could hardly believe their good fortune – after all they had gone through they were now able to enjoy the evening of their lives together in such prosperity. Even Api's wildest dreams during those dark days of 1945 had not pictured anything so bountiful. For me, a child of about 10 years, it was a perfect setting in so many ways. After all my being shuffled around where I was always a visitor with many different people, after the strict convent and the quarantine hospital, I finally felt I was home. I even had a cat, Felix, a powerful grey-striped tiger who spent the nights outside hunting. Early every morning I called for him and soon saw him bounding over the high grass of the meadow ready to share my breakfast of semolina, only he took his neat without the layer of cocoa and sugar I liberally sprinkled over mine. Then I went off to school and he slept on the couch.

The nuns' education combined with Api's steady assistance induced my elementary school to move me ahead a grade. Because of this I was not yet

9 years old when I passed the examination for the *gymnasium*, the highest level of secondary school in Germany. My new school was the Wilhelm Raabe Schule, in Lüneburg, about 25 miles away. I loved the commute by train, which I did every day with a group of friends. It felt very grown up to ride the train from the small Bevensen station into the much larger one in Lüneburg. Once there, my friends and I had a thirty-minute walk through the medieval Hanseatic city, known for its salt mines, to get to our school. It was an imposing red-brick building of the early twentieth century, so much larger than my elementary school. The broad staircases, long marble hallways and huge arched windows made me a little afraid of what was to come. The opening ceremony took place in the neo-Gothic *Aula*. I felt dwarfed by its 12ft stained-glass windows and ceiling so high I could hardly see to the top. After the all-too-easy elementary school I found the *gymnasium* very demanding. not mainly intellectually but in terms of maturity. With a birthday in October, I was almost two years younger than the rest of my classmates and, despite Api's training, not prepared for the seriousness of this education.

The curriculum started with Latin and Api worked with me on this almost every day. I still have a thick notebook which on the left side has Api's German sentences and in the right my Latin translations. I marvel today at the complexity of what he asked of me and my ability to translate. It begins with relatively easy tasks, such as 'The son jumped into the deep water of the big river and swam well'. But then it goes on to long, complicated sentences, like the following, in which I am to work out the future conditional tense:

> When you will have caught or put to flight the culprit who stole the beautiful apples from our tall apple tree, you will have been a great help not only to us but to all neighbours.

His work paid off years later when I was the only student in my MA class at Columbia to pass the Latin translation test right away. Api's tutoring, however, could not make up for the fact that at the *gymnasium* I clowned around and did not pay much attention.

When I returned from school in the afternoon Felix met me halfway on my walk home from the station, running ahead of me with a constant stream of 'meow meows'. I did not know whether he was urging me on to hurry home or whether he was just as pleased as I was to be with him. Felix was my first and only pet as a child, although 'pet' seems too frivolous a term for my serious tomcat.

56

A Visit to Bevensen

Herr Dr. Frese prescribed my first glasses.

In the winter of 2008 after Mike, Benedict and I had checked out Suderburg and Holxen, we ended the trip into my past with a visit to Bevensen. It was only a short car ride from Suderburg on narrow roads lined with birch trees, but it must have seemed long to Api on his bike. I noticed that the town no longer was simply called Bevensen, but had been given the designation of a spa. The street sign proudly proclaimed Bad Bevensen, Spa Bevensen. We looked around the flat countryside shrouded in mist and wondered how a spa could thrive here, but we soon saw that it did. The road took us directly to the spa centre which, of course, was all new to me. We saw all the usual trappings of a health resort, the park and long hall where patients walk about sipping the healthful waters. Thanks to all the moisture in the air, the grass was bright green even in winter. Beyond the public amenities was street upon street of B&Bs with names like House Barbara or House Rest. The larger establishments called themselves *Kur Hotels*, Resort Hotels. We checked into Haus Sabine for the night because I liked the birches and pines that surrounded it. It was new, modern, clean and bright, and Frau Sabine herself welcomed us. Our rooms had startlingly white lace curtains and fluffy down pillows and blankets.

As soon as we were settled, I was eager to leave this new and restful environment to show Mike and Benedict the town I knew. We took a path to the Klaubusch, the little pine wood that rises up steeply from the Ilmenau River where I used to sled, often rather dangerously, between the trees. As soon as we had descended to the river and crossed the little wooden bridge, I was back in the world of the 1950s. There were the foggy meadows of my childhood reaching up to Eckermannstrasse and the cinder path we took alongside them seemed the same as well. I thought how often I had scraped my knees bloody on the rough stones when I fell off my bike. In fact, I don't remember that my knees and shins ever were without scabs. When we came to the blue-and-white enamel sign that read Eckermannstrasse, I immediately saw that the Obstfelders' house was still there at the corner, although Api and Nyussi's arbour had gone to make way for a garden. As we walked along to No. 19, I noticed that a few of the houses had been remodelled or enlarged, but on the whole the street was much like it had been when I ran and cycled along it.

Then we stood in front of our house. It looked the same, yet also different. At first I could not pinpoint what had changed but then I saw that an entire wing had been added on the side where Nyussi's winter garden used to be. The two entrances, however, were the same, and the present owners still used one for business and one for living. Now instead of a surgery, the right entrance led to Sommer Accounting Services. I went up to the office and rang the bell. Herr Sommer Senior himself opened the door. I explained who I was and he let me in. We walked through the waiting room to his office, Api's former surgery. Herr Sommer told me that he remembered Dr Frese: 'In 1953 he prescribed me my first glasses.' I was surprised and happy that there still was just a little connection to Api in this house. When Herr Sommer showed me around, I saw that most rooms had been remodelled. Nevertheless, there were still touches left that, with a surge in my heart, brought me back to my childhood: brass door handles that I had long forgotten but now remembered; the two sets of stairs I had run up and down so often, the main one going up from Nyussi's winter garden and the other from Api's office. Even the living room looking out on the veranda was much like it used to be. After I said goodbye to Herr Sommer, I could not stop talking about it all to Mike and Benedict, especially that Herr Sommer had remembered Api.

From the house we took a walk into town. The path now was paved and houses lined one side of it, but on the other the view across a misty meadow to the church was exactly the same. When we reached the main street, there still was the bakery where I used to buy *Bienenstich*, a yeast, custard and nut confection we all loved. Of course, the three of us needed to stop and each have a slice. Then I showed them the way to the station that I had taken every day. Again I was astonished how little had changed, and that even many of the businesses had remained the same. I pointed out each new find. There was the paper store, Schliekau, where I got my exercise books and where Api had bought me my first fountain pen, a green Pelikan of which I was very proud. At the corner where we turned into Bahnhofstrasse I spotted the tobacconist store, Harms, where Api had purchased his cigars. Then we came to the park, also the same, and beyond it lay the station square. The station building had two wings, each with three tall, curved windows. The middle section was higher and had the same set of windows, one above the other. Steps led into the station hall. It must have been rather large for what then was a small town where the express trains did not stop. I ran up the steps ahead of Mike and Benedict to find the station hall and the platforms just as I remembered them. I could have been rushing to catch the train to Lüneburg.

On our way back to Haus Sabine we headed for the Church of the Epiphany, which I had attended every Sunday with Api and Nyussi. I thought of our walks there in any weather, of Api's asking me about the sermon afterwards and of the wonderful *Siebenstern* service on Christmas Eve. We passed through a short, tree-lined avenue to reach the church, which is dominated by its high, pointed steeple. The interior was simple but more beautiful than I remembered it. The plain white walls bore golden decorations around the windows and the seat cushions in the pews were a rich red. The altar was decorated with a motif of grapes and ears of grain. I remembered that Api had told me that the site once housed a church dating back to the year 833, but that a fire had destroyed it at the beginning of the nineteenth century, after which this church was erected. At Haus Sabine we ended the day with a game of *Halma*, pickup sticks, which we found in the lounge. Api and I had often played that game, although Api was always more patient and his hand, used to delicate eye operations, steadier than mine.

At night I kept thinking about Api. I realised, more strongly perhaps than before, that so many years later his values still are with me. I have adopted his love of nature and his commitment to single-minded work and play. To this day I do not like to watch television or even listen to music while working or reading. Even now, when I am older than Api, I still love games of all sorts and get a childlike enjoyment from playing. My emotional, often sentimental attitude also stems from him and he himself was well aware of his sentimental tendencies. These often show themselves in his diaries, as when he thinks back nostalgically to his past and finds himself unable to leave his Luisenstrasse apartment because of the happy memories associated with it, or when he waxes emotional about his new refuge, the little 'swallow's nest'. I may even outdo my grandfather in sentimentality, such as my 'friends' on the road. On routes I travel frequently I have chosen some object, such as the mileage marker 270 on the way to my stepfather in Urbana, or a red-and-white-striped smokestack, 'power and light', on the southern outskirts of Indianapolis and I greet my 'friends' whenever I travel past them.

I was grateful that Mike and Benedict were with me on this journey. As I drifted off to sleep, I thought how gratefulness for what I have was another trait Api had instilled in me, how I was especially grateful for all he had done for me, the love he had shown me and, finally, I hoped that this book would not displease him.

57

Gloves at the Bottom of the Stairs

Farewell, be happy. Only in parting are we truly one.

Unfortunately, Api had such a very short time to enjoy all he had achieved after the war. He lived just over two years in his new home. At midnight on New Year's Eve 1954 I recited the poem for that year as I had done each year I lived with him. Api always gave me the poem well ahead of time so that I could memorise it and he coached me in its presentation. It was our secret and no one else in the family heard the poem before the event.

Api gave me the poem for New Year's Eve 1954/55 right after Christmas. As in all the previous years, I copied it out so that today I have both Api's version and mine in my rounded childish script. I had the poem memorised a few days later and we worked on it together when no one was around to hear us. Little did I know that this would be the last time we did this together. Today, the poem reads like a premonition of his death eleven days later. It certainly is a farewell, although I am not sure that either Nyussi or my mother, who had joined us from Vienna, saw it as anything else than a metaphor for bidding the old year goodbye:

New Year's Eve 1954
An old man wanders slow and quiet through the street
Where for a year he intimately lived with us
Worked, suffered, laughed. Prepared now to retreat,
Just checking whether it's been good.
Troubled I watch him leave, with almost tearful eye
Perhaps he notices and takes it as it's meant
A silent thanks. I see his grey head bow, then he is gone:
Farewell, be happy. Only in parting are we truly one.

I wonder whether when Api composed that last line he was hearing a faint echo of those months in 1945 when, at his most desperate moments, he consoled himself with the idea of a reunion in God? Was he now again taking refuge in this sentiment because of a premonition of death?

Api died suddenly in the night of 11/12 January 1955 of a massive heart attack, less than two weeks before his sixty-seventh birthday. As I was writing this I recognised with a shock that this is a year younger than I am now. He had just managed to drive himself back from Kloster Medingen, where he had visited and tended to his aged friends in the county retirement home. The old men in the home always looked forward to Api's visits, not only for the eye care but for the laughter and joy he brought into their quiet lives. Api also enjoyed their company and looked after them for free. I often had accompanied him on these visits on Saturday afternoons, following in his wake of laughter and jokes. But this time he went alone after work in the evening when I was already in bed. Late at night I heard some unusual commotion, but did not find out that Api had died until the next morning.

It was the first time in my life that I had consciously come close to death and it took me a long time to understand that I would never be with Api again. What I remember from the next morning was seeing his gloves lying at the bottom of the stairs that led up to the bedroom from his surgery. Api never left his things lying about. He had discarded them hastily the night before when he was trying to reach his bed before collapsing. The fingers of the gloves were still bent from his hand but they looked rigid, dead. For days afterwards I saw the gloves whenever I passed the stairs for no one took them away. The image of the gloves with the bent fingers came to me in dreams for years after Api's death.

Api's body was laid out in the sun room, next to Nyussi's red and purple cyclamens. Many people came to say their goodbyes. When no one was there I stood by his body, noticing that his fingernails had turned violet blue, but not really grasping that this was my Api lying there in his formal dark-blue pin-striped suit. In fact, sometimes I rushed into the room not even remembering that Api was there. That rigid body just could not be him.

Nyussi had put Api's death notice under the motto of 'We dwell like those who always have to migrate'. It is a translation from the Latin '*tanquam migraturi habitamus*', but I do not know from where. It seems to fit us all.

We received mountains of flowers for the funeral. In the short time he was there, Api had been loved and respected by the people of Bevensen. He was put to rest in the small Bevensen cemetery with the heather bushes and birch trees he had come to love keeping him company. The headstone was a simple field stone such as dotted the heath all around us. It reminded me of the medieval church tower in Suderburg. His friend, Superintendent Stünkel, gave the eulogy, but I don't remember a single word he said. It all still was not real to me. It is only over the years that I have understood that I will mourn Api all my life. He was my anchor and I will always miss his unconditional love. Although I cannot share his idea that only in parting are we truly one, over the years I have come to appreciate how much of his spirit has remained with me and has become part of me.

Our final stop in Bevensen in 2008 was the cemetery. When I stood at Api's grave, I suddenly began to cry, overcome by a feeling of childish abandonment. But then my husband and son stood by me and I felt their love and sought refuge in their presence and support.

After Api's death life changed dramatically for both Nyussi and me. My mother had come back from Vienna but she went on to Hamburg, where she studied to become a business school teacher as her father had wished. Nyussi and I were alone in the house. Nyussi had been advised to rent out the practice until we knew better what to do. The eye doctor we took in to run the practice and live with us turned out to be a morphine addict. He wandered about at night, the pupils of his eyes huge and black, talking fantastically. We hid from him whenever possible. I still ate my morning porridge with Felix the cat and went off on the train each morning, but I began to fail in school. In less than a year it became clear that Nyussi and

I were unable to handle the situation. She sold the practice and the house for much less than it was worth, and in the summer of 1956 I once again was back at a boarding school, this time on the Baltic Sea, and repeated the grade I had just finished.

In his diaries Api had written about how helpless and distraught he was without us, how he needed us. Without us, he felt unable to make any decisions and was barely able to survive. After his death we saw how much our lives were based on his planning and provisions, how defenceless we were without him and how much we needed him. For me, Api's death abruptly brought an end to the five happiest years of my childhood. Nyussi survived her husband by only three years during which time, although increasingly ill, she was my strongest support.

As I grew to be a teenager and discovered an interest in my schoolwork, Api began to be with and within me. After failing in school during the year after his death, I excelled in my work and became ambitious and committed to study and learn more. I then remembered what he had told me so often and tried to live up to his rule of work before play, and to do both, work or play, wholeheartedly, giving it my full attention. I enjoyed listening to classical music, as he had done. He would be pleased to know that now I, too, would have chosen Verdi over an operetta. Api had been the only father figure I had known and I cherished his memory, his love and his *joie de vivre*. Even as I grew to be an adult he remained my role model, but it never was a stern and rigid image I had of him, rather one filled with gladness and good spirits. He taught me to be grateful for whatever I have and enjoy every moment. I still feel free to preserve a childlike glee about the little things in life as he had done. Even today, at age 67, I am not beyond skipping along the street when I am feeling good. Api taught me to love nature, and, yes, to wax sentimental at times. When I did well at the university, won a Woodrow Wilson Fellowship and received my PhD at the age of 25, I imagined him watching me succeed and approve and be proud of what I had accomplished.

Then at the end of my career I found the diary. First I was surprised how fearful and helpless Api had been in Berlin in 1945. I still had the child's image of a strong father who was never at a loss of what to do. Reading his words made me feel closer to him, understanding him not as my grandfather Api but as a man on his own, loving and so very vulnerable. I began to think about what I knew of his life before he became my grandfather, his Prussian upbringing, which explained many of the beliefs and mental bearings he had instilled also in me. Over a gulf of sixty years, I felt closer to Api than ever before.

Then I discovered that Api had been a Nazi. It was a physical shock. I had lived more than thirty years in the United States and absorbed the image of the cold-blooded, steely eyed and cruel Nazi as he is portrayed again and again in films and stories. How could Api be one of them? I could not answer that question but resolved that I would keep his secret.

When Mike at last persuaded me to write Api's story after all, I had to confront the issue of his Nazi Party membership. Learning more about that time and Api's circumstances helped me to explain and understand, although it did not answer all questions. I often was reminded of Edward Ball's account of the slaves in his family and, like him, hoped that by recounting Api's story, I would not 'dig up my grandfather and hang him', but instead come closer both to him and to some sense of accountability.

58

Trying to Understand

May the Almighty God take our work into His
mercy, form our will justly, bless our understanding
and gladden us with the trust of our people.

L
ooking back, I have to admit that this recounting and accounting
has left many of the questions with which I set out and which have
kept cropping up all along unanswered. How can I account for
Api's Nazi membership and how can I assess his individual guilt
during the years of the Nazi terror?

Api was formed by his small-town Prussian upbringing at the end of the
nineteenth century. The years of his military service reinforced the lessons
of discipline and obedience to authority he had learnt from his family and
in school. He was always proud to wear his uniform and proud, too, of his
country. He was raised as a conservative and remained so all his life. Coming
out of the First World War, Api was bewildered and at odds with the world
into which he was thrown. The abdication of the emperor was a blow to
his Prussian sensibilities, and there was no one to fill that void. The Weimar
Republic under President Ebert was never strong enough to assert itself
against the extremists on both the Right and the Left. Ebert's attempts at
a pro-democratic government were drowned in a cacophony of violence.
Although Api prospered economically in the 1920s, he did not subscribe to

the ethos of the roaring twenties with its emancipated women, biting wit, stark expressionist art, social revolutionary spirit and sexual liberation. He never made the transition into this new world.

The golden twenties did not last long, either. The stock market crash of 1929 triggered another economic crisis. By 1932, Germany had 6.1 million unemployed. Banks collapsed and the stock market had to be closed for more than a month. Politically, the situation was no more stable. Rival political gangs kept fighting and even murdering each other and there were a total of five elections that year, none of them conclusive. Seeing all this, Api must have feared that the newly won order and prosperity would disintegrate once more, as it had after the war.

When Api joined the Nazi Party on 1 May 1933 he may well have seen Hitler as the best hope for a battered Germany and believed his promises of stability, peace and Christian values. With the political weakness of the Weimar government on one side, and the threat of international communism on the other, Api may have appreciated Hitler as a man strong enough to stand up against all the forever-warring parties. Api perfectly fit the profile of Hitler's supporters in the early 1930s. They tended to be older, conservative, Protestant and anti-socialist or anti-communist.

Strangely enough, even Api's religious faith may have helped to incline him towards Hitler. From childhood on, Api was steeped in a pietistic Lutheranism, a religion of the heart that thrived on introspection and a study of the Bible. It taught him to be tolerant, modest and compassionate, but it also made a clear distinction between private and public life, allowing the two spheres to exist independently side by side. In his 1946 book, *The Solution of the German Question*, Wilhelm Röpke, a political, economic and social theorist, argued that this Lutheranism which makes a sharp distinction between the political and public outer world and man's own soul helped to pave the way for the Nazi regime:

> The two are entirely separate from each other, and thus demand quite different conduct; they may even be ruled by opposite moral principles without disturbing each other ... Thus this doctrine meant for the Germans a school of non-resistance against the power of the state, of political indifference ... and of submission to the authorities in all questions of public life.

Moreover, at the start Hitler presented himself as a deeply religious man. He wove into his speeches constant references to God's blessing, Christian ethics and even ended them with 'Amen'. Thus on 1 February 1933, he assured his listeners that Christianity was his foundation, concluding with: 'May the almighty God take our work into His mercy, form our will justly, bless our understanding and gladden us with the trust of our people.' Bishop Dibelius, who had officiated on the Day of Potsdam, wrote that there will be few pastors who will not be heartily glad of this new direction initiated by Hitler. Together with most members of German National Protestantism, Api must have thought that Hitler would preside over a new Christian state.

In trying to come closer to why Api joined the Party, I also reminded myself that in 1933 the National Socialists 'were popular in so far as they were identified with a new national mood that emphasised national integration, social reform, and economic prosperity'. Hitler came to power legally, not through a coup or revolution. According to George Mosse, a historian of racism and nationalism, that in itself turned fatal for many moderate voters like my grandfather:

> If there had been barricades instead of legality in 1933, men and women would have been forced to make more reasoned decisions. The legal assumption of power, however, allowed them to drift into the open arms of the Third Reich, finding themselves in an embrace from which there was no escape, except prison or exile.

The Nazis promised both cultural and social regeneration, which appealed to my grandfather who had been dismayed by what he considered the collapse of traditional values in the 1920s. Early on Hitler said nothing about exterminating Jews or enslaving Russians. In fact his speeches in the early 1930s tended to promote moderation and stress his peaceful intentions. On 16 March 1935, when he had just instituted compulsory military service, Hitler assured everyone in Germany and beyond: 'The government of today's Germany desires only a single moral and material power: it is the power to preserve peace for the Reich and therefore also for all of Europe.' Therefore, historian MacDonogh argues, 'To make all Germans responsible for the relatively docile Hitler of 1933 is to apply the Allied weapon of collective guilt.'

59

And Yet …

If Goldhagen is right about the uniquely German cause of the Holocaust, the rest of us need never again say, 'Never again!'

Yet astute and aware political observers could, and did have, some idea of Hitler's true nature and aims, even in the early 1930s. He had published *Mein Kampf* in 1925 in which he outlined many of the ideas he was to realise through war and violence when he came to power. His book proclaims his racist worldview, his anti-Semitism, hatred of communism and the need of the 'master race' for more *Lebensraum*, space for life. The writer Erich Ebermayer is an example of a person who acknowledged Hitler's moderate and statesmanlike behaviour immediately after 1933, and yet refused to be taken in by these gestures of apparent good will. At most, Ebermayer expressed the ardent hope that Hitler would be as good as his word. But at heart Ebermayer never doubted that Hitler was blatantly lying. For there were also signs in Hitler's speeches and especially in the rhetoric of Joseph Goebbels, his Reich Minister of Public Enlightenment and Propaganda, that should have made Api refuse to vote for a man who more than any other politician or movement stood against everything he held dear.

I also know that Hitler created neither his racist ideology nor his territorial expansion out of thin air, but built on existing German prejudices and longings, especially among conservatives. I have to ask myself if Api shared either in the racism or in the desire for *Lebensraum*, or both. He may well have wanted Germany to regain the part of Prussia that now was Poland. He, after all, grew up there. Could his silence in the diaries about the persecution of the Jews be any indication of anti-Semitism? I do not like to jump to this conclusion but have to admit that I just do not know.

In the end I cannot get around the fact that Germans who voted for Hitler or joined the Party bear a responsibility, even if, like Api, after joining the Party they took no further part in any of its activities. That responsibility lies perhaps heaviest not only on Api personally but on his class of educated professionals who should have known better and not given in so easily to Hitler's lure. That is why Peter Fritsche concluded in 1998: 'The brutal terms in which all nationalists regarded the enemies of Germany and the correspondingly imperious way they defined its future made most Germans complicit in the crimes of Nazism.'

This is similar to the thesis of Daniel Jonah Goldhagen's haunting book *Hitler's Willing Executioners: Ordinary Germans and the Holocaust.* It claims that Germans acted out of a century-old eliminationist anti-Semitism and demonstrates the ubiquity of anti-Semitism in the Germany of that time. Reading this, I have to ask myself once again whether, or to what degree, Api had been affected by this prevailing prejudice. Goldhagen finds strong anti-Semitic bias at all levels of German society from aristocrats to workers, soldiers, professionals and members of industry. Anti-Semitism was everywhere; in all parts of the country from Bavaria in the south to Api's beloved Prussia in the north-east. Goldhagen claims that their statements prove that as late as 1944 even the members of the 20 July plot to assassinate Hitler shared the Führer's anti-Semitism. It also was rampant, he argues, in the Protestant Church, where it was widespread among the clergy from pastors to bishops, and showed itself clearly in Church publications, such as the weekly *Sonntagsblätter*, Sunday leaflets. He indicts even the Protestant theologian Karl Barth and the Lutheran Pastor Dietrich Bonhoeffer, whom Hitler executed in 1945. Goldhagen blames the character of the German people as a whole. He paints Germans as different from all other civilised people in that they have been obsessed with 'eliminationist' anti-Semitism for more than a hundred years. This enabled them to participate in the Nazi regime and its anti-Semitism and made them capable of genocide.

These are damning allegations, but I reminded myself that Goldhagen's assertions have been hotly contested both here and abroad. Scholars like A.C. Grayling, Omer Bartov, Clive James and Richard Neuhaus have testified to the questionable character of Goldhagen's scholarship. Neuhaus finds much to criticise about Goldhagen's thesis, such as the way it misrepresents German pre-Nazi history and ignores the realities that prevented effective German resistance. Neuhaus also takes issue with Goldhagen's view of the German churches as eager members of Hitler's willing executioners: 'It is simply not true to say that the churches welcomed the ascendancy of the Nazis.' Writing seven years before Goldhagen, historian Hans Mommsen claims that there were not more than 20 per cent active anti-Semites in the ranks of the NSDAP and that only the conditions of war with Russia allowed the Nazis to put the 'final solution' into action. Above all, scholars have rejected Goldhagen's attempt to keep alive the notion of the collective guilt of the Germans who are unlike the rest of the world. In fact, they see such a view as highly dangerous since it nullifies the moral significance of the Holocaust: 'If Goldhagen is right about the uniquely German cause of the Holocaust, the rest of us need never again say, "Never again"!'

Moreover, who, either in Germany or abroad, could have been prepared for a man like Hitler? Sebastian Haffner writes about this: 'Our thinking is usually constrained by a certain civilization in our outlook, in which the basics are unquestioned ... certain Christian, humanistic, civilized principles [are accepted] as axiomatic.' Hannah Arendt said that only a madman could have predicted what was coming. She believes that 'they, [and she includes not only Germans but other nations] who were the Nazis' first accomplices and their best aids, truly did not know what they were doing and with whom they were dealing'. These sentiments are echoed by Peter Gay, an emigrant from Nazi Germany who became professor at Yale University with an interest in the social history of ideas. Gay wrote in his memoir of 1998: 'Hitler's threats were so utterly implausible that we regarded them as unreliable guides to future conduct.' Peter Gay was born Peter Föhlich into a Jewish family in Berlin. They did not flee Berlin until 1938 and he was shocked when Jews in America battered him with hostile questions as to why his family had not emigrated much earlier.

During the first five years of Hitler's rule the world at large was not denouncing Hitler or standing up against him either. Quite the contrary. In July 1933 the Vatican signed an agreement, a Papal Concordat, with Hitler, which helped to give him legitimacy in Germany and abroad. The papal endorsement also removed the Catholic Church in Germany from any serious opposition to Hitler. In 1936 Hitler occupied the Rhineland, but France did nothing. Even in the later 1930s no other than Winston Churchill, although not blind to Hitler's ruthlessness, nevertheless found words of praise for him. In his 1935 article 'Hitler and His Choice' for *The Strand*, reprinted in his 1937 book *Great Contemporaries*, Churchill wrote:

> While all those formidable transformations were occurring in Europe, Corporal Hitler was fighting his long, wearing battle for the German heart. The story of that battle cannot be read without admiration for the courage, the perseverance, and the vital force which enabled him to challenge, defy, conciliate, or overcome, all the authorities or resistances which barred his path.

At the end of the essay Churchill said: 'Those who have met Herr Hitler face to face in public business or on social terms have found a highly competent, cool, well-informed functionary with an agreeable manner, a disarming smile, and few have been unaffected by a subtle personal magnetism.' Two years later, in an article of 17 September 1937 (published in *Step by Step* in 1939) Churchill said further: 'One may dislike Hitler's system and yet admire his patriotic achievement. If our country were defeated, I hope we should find a champion as indomitable to restore our courage and lead us back to our place among the nations.' Both Karl Japers and Wilhelm Roepke remember that as late as 1938 Churchill published an open letter to Hitler in the *London Times*, which said among other things: 'Were England to suffer a national disaster comparable to that of Germany in 1918, I should pray to God to send us a man of your strength of mind and will.' Journalists Adam LeBor and Roger Boyes also indict the British upper classes, including King Edward VIII. They saw widespread support for Hitler among the financial, political and industrial Establishment of Great Britain.

Otto Friedrich sums up this international support for Hitler and its effect on Berliners:

> For the Berliners of those early years, it must have seemed that Hitler not only achieved great successes but won the praise of the outside world ... When Hitler cancelled all reparations, when Hitler marched troops into the Rhineland, when Hitler walked out of the League of Nations, when Hitler staged the *Anschluss* with Austria – which of the great powers of the world did anything to stop him? And what lessons should the ordinary Berliner have drawn from Hitler's triumphs?

60

Inner Emigration

I myself was to experience how easily one is taken
in by a lying and censored press and radio in a
totalitarian state.

In an effort to try to come to grips with this troubling and perplexing
question of Api's guilt, I sought counsel from other testimonies of
the time by people who lived through the same conditions. Writing
from Nazi Germany, journalist William Shirer noted the effect of
living under a totalitarian regime: 'No one who has not lived for years in a
totalitarian land can possibly conceive how difficult it is to escape the dread
consequences of a regime's calculated and incessant propaganda.' Shirer
admits that, 'I myself was to experience how easily one is taken in by a lying
and censored press and radio in a totalitarian state'. Unlike most Germans,
Shirer had access to foreign newspapers and radio broadcasts. Despite this
he felt that 'it was surprising and sometimes consternating to find that
notwithstanding the opportunities I had to learn the facts and despite one's
inherent distrust of what one learned from Nazi sources, a steady diet over
the years of falsifications and distortions made a certain impression on
one's mind and often misled it'.

Looking back on the Third Reich from the perspective of the twenty-
first century, historian Tobias Jersak sees a related effect of Hitler's

propaganda: 'The first norm which Hitler and his followers changed was logic itself: they did so by introducing a *new* logic, i.e. new rules of right thinking.' It created profound self-doubt in the individual, 'This self-doubt consisted precisely in doubting the rightness of one's own thinking. And when that is in question, active protest is impossible.' Jersak's formulation made me think of Api's almost paralysing self-doubt throughout the months of 1945 and I wondered whether this was not alone the result of his immediate situation but had been building during the years of the Nazi regime.

Mathilde Wolff-Mönckeberg lived under the Nazis and later wrote about her experience. She was a member of one of the foremost families in Hamburg – a main shopping street is named Mönckebergstrasse after her family. Her husband was a professor at the university and a senator, which is a most prestigious position in the twelve-member Cabinet of the Free and Hanseatic City of Hamburg. Hamburg, always close to Great Britain, altogether had been one of the cities least prone to Nazi propaganda. My stepfather, who went to school in Hamburg since 1935, remembers that he never had a Nazi teacher nor was he lectured on race education and other matters of the Nazi curriculum. After the war, Mathilde Wolff-Mönckeberg was much troubled by this issue of guilt. Her book about her experiences, titled *On the Other Side*, is dedicated to her children to whom she is trying to explain what it was like to live under the Nazis. She had not been a member of the Party and had been disgusted with the regime all along. However, after the war, when Hamburg was under British occupation, the British officers with whom she talked believed that all Germans were equally responsible for the atrocities of the Nazi regime. She tried in vain to make them understand that neither she nor her husband could have done anything: 'It was totally impossible to form an opposition, spied upon as we were from all sides, telephone conversations listened in to, people standing behind us and alongside us listening and denouncing. It would have cost us our lives, or we should have ended up in concentration camps.'

The doctor and poet Gottfried Benn, who like Api had been educated at the Emperor Wilhelm Military Academy and served as doctor in both world wars, wrote from Berlin in a letter of 19 March 1945: 'He who wants to talk and judge Germany must have stayed here.' Theodor Heuss, who in 1949 was to become the first elected President of the Federal Republic of

Germany, similarly said after the war that 'only he who has lived twelve years under the Nazi terror can judge how enormous this pressure was and how much heroism and political insight were required to resist it'. He was trying to urge restraint in American de-Nazification procedures. Even if such statements as Benn's and Heuss' sound a little self-serving or one-sided, they give one pause about easy judgements and categorical and unilateral condemnation.

I well remember a phrase that was much used after the war. It was *innere Emigration*, inner emigration. I often caught those words as my grandparents listened to the radio, although I had no idea what they meant. Germans now claimed that they had not supported Hitler's brutal regime but since they were powerless to act against it, and since they were unable to leave the country, their only option was withdrawal or 'inner emigration'. It has indeed been observed that after 1933 many people, Api and his family among them, withdrew from politics and public demonstrations and instead focused all their energies on their families and their private lives. Not only apolitical people like Api engaged in this, but 'even politically-minded people withdrew into privacy in face of the constant pressure to conform, the perpetual need to demonstrate loyalty, the thought control and the bureaucratic routine that marked public life under National Socialism'. This may well have been an inner emigration. Yet again it also seems too easy an excuse, a willed and partial blindness to what was going on around them. In the end, inner emigration entails a passive consent and acceptance of Nazi atrocities. Therefore, the notion of inner emigration has been widely criticised as just another way Germans were evading their responsibility.

The philosopher Karl Jaspers, who lived in Germany during the war, faced this responsibility squarely. Writing in 1946, he stated without prevarication that, 'we Germans, every German, is guilty in some way'. He rephrased this notion repeatedly. At one point he noted: 'In view of the crimes which were committed in the name of the Reich, each German is co-responsible. We are all collectively liable.' But Jaspers also recognised the limits of this political responsibility:

Germany under the Nazi regime was a penitentiary. The guilt of getting into this penitentiary is political guilt. But once the gates had fallen shut, it became impossible to break out of this penitentiary

295

from within. Any discussion of what responsibility and guilt of the imprisoned remains and arises thereafter must consider the question what under such circumstances they can do at all.

Jaspers found all Germans, himself included, guilty not only politically but also morally and metaphysically. Everyone in Hitler's Germany made some gestures of accommodation; they may have attended meetings and rallies, given the Hitler salute saying '*Heil Hitler*' or, faced with threatening bodies like the Gestapo, pretended loyalty. 'We did not go into the streets when our Jewish friends were led away; we did not scream out until we, too, were destroyed. We preferred to stay alive on the feeble, if correct, ground that our death could not have helped in any way. The fact that we live, that is our guilt.'

If we accept Jaspers' uncompromising view of political responsibility, we are all implicated and politically responsible for the acts of our government. Jaspers acknowledges this: 'Politically everyone acts in the modern state, at least by voting, or failing to vote, in elections. The sense of political liability leaves no one a way out.' Api, a member of the Nazi Party, was responsible. By that argument, however, so are we if we allow our government to engage in torture and war or, even closer to home, stand by when we know racism and social injustice to destroy lives around us. We become guilty just by being silent bystanders.

However, to avoid painting with too broad a brush Jaspers makes clear that this responsibility is an individual matter and has to be considered carefully case by case. Otherwise, the very notion of guilt and responsibility becomes meaningless. Jaspers, therefore, gauged this liability not collectively but saw the degree of guilt as different for each individual. When and why someone joined the Party, how they supported the regime, what even small acts of resistance they risked in their daily lives – all have to be taken into account. Between the extremes of murdering people in concentration camps and risking one's life by hiding Jewish friends, there were so very many degrees of choice for everyone.

As I ponder this, I am nagged by questions about what I would have done: how far would I have been willing to adapt, to go along, to commit small acts of cowardice and submission? Like Api, I am not particularly politically interested or engaged, and could easily have become as withdrawn into my private world and ready to compromise as he seemed to have done. Similar questions have troubled many people of my post-war generation. As one writer puts it, 'In how far can a human being be sure of her or himself?'

In her 1945 essay 'Organized Guilt and Universal Responsibility', Hannah Arendt made a similar argument that the measure of guilt 'can be determined only by the One who knows the secrets of the human heart, which no human eye can penetrate'. Arendt, who fled Nazi Germany first to France and then in 1941 to the United States, had grown up in Königsberg, Prussia and Berlin, and had written her dissertation under Karl Jaspers. She went on to say that 'where all are guilty, nobody in the last analysis can be judged'. Arendt distinguishes between guilt and responsibility, saying that 'there are many who share responsibility without any visible proof of guilt'. She includes in this group leaders from other countries and ultimately every human being. 'For the idea of humanity, when purged of all sentimentality, has the very serious consequence that in one form or another men must assume responsibility for all crimes committed by men and that all nations share the onus of evil committed by all others.' The Jewish genocide entails the crisis of our humanity and our morality.

Wilhelm Röpke, who by no means excused the Germans for the crimes of the Nazis, also fights the idea of collective guilt: 'The thesis of the collective guilt of all Germans, which served as an excuse for the worst blunders of the Allies in Germany, could have been posthumously invented by Dr. Goebbels.' In his view, blaming an entire nation implies a betrayal of the principle of personal responsibility, a cornerstone of our civilisation, in favour of a collectivist notion that eliminates individuality.

Observers have noted that at the end of the war most Germans were like my grandfather and did not reflect on their national guilt. The Reverend David Cairns, member of a Scottish regiment, told a meeting of the British Council of Churches that German civilians were obsessed with their own survival and that of their families and friends. He was particularly bothered by 'the lack of understanding for the suffering that Germany has caused other people'. In his estimation, the sense of guilt was 'rather lacking'. General Lucius Clay, who had been Eisenhower's deputy and after the war was military governor of the US zone of Germany, voiced the same sentiment: 'The German masses seem totally apolitical, apathetic and primarily concerned with everyday problems of food, shelter and clothing ... No general feeling of war guilt or repugnance for Nazi doctrine and regime has manifested itself. Germans blame Nazis for losing war, protest ignorance of the regime's crimes and shrug off their own support as incidental and unavoidable.'

General Clay's summary of German attitudes rings true, even if expressed without much sympathy. Lack of sympathy for Germans is, of course, understandable right at the end of a war which had cost the lives of millions of Allies. Yet it does not seem quite as surprising as these observers thought that, during a time when they lived through an inferno, had lost many members of their families and their own survival was in doubt, Germans did not dwell on the problem of collective guilt. As Jaspers noted concerning that large part of the population who existed without home, work and bread: 'The horizon has become narrow. One does not want to hear about guilt, about the past. One is not concerned about world history. One simply wants the suffering to cease.'

I can also imagine that it was not only their own suffering that made people apathetic. The deaths of millions of people – soldiers in the field, women and children in cities and towns, 0.25 million civilians during the atom bomb attacks on Japan and 6 million in concentration camps – had been too much to take in and effectively deadened people's imagination and feelings.

I cannot measure if and to what extent Api, individually, is politically responsible, even if he himself felt innocent. Given that doubt, should we then discount his suffering because of this guilt or even see it as just deserts? Or should we discount it because others suffered even worse? This makes me think of the article by Columbia Professor Mark M. Anderson, which helped me to overcome my reluctance to get started with this recounting of Api's story. Anderson said that after the war 'German victimhood became politically incorrect'. More recently, however, with the passing of the generation that lived through the war, that is beginning to change. 'Unacknowledged suffering claims its due' and 'individual suffering, not a simple tallying of perpetrators and victims, is beginning to emerge in striking historical detail and complexity'. This by no means implies a lessening of the horror and unexceeded brutality of the Holocaust. Instead, Anderson concludes, stories of German war experiences tell us 'the importance of individual historical experience that resists the either/or of victimhood. In a sense, arguing over whose victims can be counted is another way of continuing the war – a war that may truly be over only when we stop feeling the need to deny the Germans their stories of suffering and loss.'

Api's individual historical experience has value to us without in any way reducing that of millions of victims of the Nazi regime. Perhaps that experience can help us to understand not only the past but to assess our present situation more clearly and make us each feel, if not responsible, at least accountable for what happens around us. Understanding experiences like my grandfather's may temper accountability with compassion, and perhaps it might help to build a future free of such horrors.

A general discussion along these lines is carried on in the twenty-first century with renewed intensity. The titles of two recent books demonstrate the contrasting positions at their most extreme. *A People of Murderers?* (1997) is a response to Goldhagen's book and *A People of Victims?* (2003) addresses historian Jörg Friedrich's *The Fire*, which describes the bombing of German cities. Murderers or victims? Some third-generation Germans, the grandchildren of those who lived at that time, suggest that it is the silence which the war generation so adamantly maintained all their lives that changes them from victims to perpetrators.

61

A Wide Field

That is a wide field, Louise.

And yet, and yet ... the questions still won't go away. Layers and layers of them keep ricocheting in my mind compelling me to go over the same ground again and again. I cannot forget the living hell of Api's daily struggle for survival in Berlin; the inferno of flames and smoke and the stench of corpses. Api lost his only son, his livelihood and his home. He was surrounded by people dying from hunger and illness, or just from weakness and, despite being a doctor, he could do so little to help them. He was alone and homeless and persecuted like a criminal.

In 1933 he became a member of the Nazi Party and continued his successful career under Hitler's regime. Yet he had established most of it, his practice and apartment in the premier medical district of Berlin, even his eight-cylinder Buick, well before the Nazis took over. His success was achieved by his Prussian values of hard work and thrift. He started out poor and it took him years to buy his instruments and furnish his practice and his apartment. He sent his family on holidays and himself stayed in Berlin to keep his office running. Nevertheless, in the 1930s his Party membership helped him to prosper in a way he would not have done without it.

Api was a member of the Nazi Party and did not revolt against the regime, but no other member of his family was a Party member. It was, therefore, not a matter of family conviction. I am certain – and his de-Nazification document which lists him as Exonerated confirms this – that he himself maintained his personal integrity, but he tried to do so outside of politics. One could argue that at a time when your country is engaged in unparalleled atrocities, there is guilt in trying to live outside politics. It means that one has to turn a blind eye, even if most of us would not have done otherwise. In 1945 Api did voice regret at his inaction, but at the same time he felt that there was nothing else he could have done. He saw himself as 'well knowing but impotent'.

During Hitler's totalitarian regime Api focused on the circle of his immediate family and as a doctor he dedicated his life to helping people. This is also how I knew Api. In Bevensen in the 1950s he looked after people in an old folks' home for free and at his death many of his patients came forward who were grateful for what Api had done for them. From earlier times I have only one personal account from a woman who wrote that her life would have been sadder and poorer had it not been for the care Dr Frese had given her. Api had treated her from 1928 to 1944 and then she looked him up again in Bevensen after the war. Although, she said, he was known as one of the best eye doctors in Berlin, he took the time to befriend her. In times of trouble he was almost like a second father to her. I do not know the specific circumstances of her case but I am pleased that this woman's testimony confirmed my sense of my grandfather.

Of course, without trying to become an apologist for his actions or lack of action, my judgement inevitably is influenced by my love for my grandfather who, in the 1950s, gave me the only home I knew up to then. He was already in his sixties and had to start all over again for himself and his wife. Nonetheless, he took me in without hesitation and looked after me, loved me, educated me, brought joy into my life and always was a secure and affectionate presence. So I am not able to judge Api. He was battered by history, one of the almost uniquely unfortunate in a generation that had to see service in two world wars and endure a frightening and brutal totalitarian regime.

Overwhelmed, I take refuge in old von Briest's response to his bewildering world in Theodor Fontane's novel of 1894, the very work behind which

I discovered the diaries. Whenever he was confronted with the fearful complexities of his life, Briest shrugged his shoulders in helpless resignation and said to his wife: 'That is a wide field, Louise.' In this way he avoided becoming judgemental of a world he no longer understood. Old Briest firmly belonged to the nineteenth-century world of the Prussian *Junker*. He was part of that landed gentry whose conservatism dominated both the Prussian civil service and the military. The end of the century, however, brought social and cultural changes which were antithetical to the straightforward *Junker* tradition in which Briest was raised. Yet he does not judge or condemn a world so different from the one he holds dear. He does not get caught up in heated arguments or fanatically defend his position. He simply lives his life in private, independent of the new ethos of his times. Old Briest's wide field expresses an at once sensitive understanding of the fatalities and irresolvable dilemmas of life and a sad resignation to understand them. The only thing he will not question or give up is his love for his family, including or even especially for his 'fallen' daughter Effie.

Perhaps the intimate details of Api's life also are such a wide field. They allow a glimpse into the fate of his generation churned up by 'the almost uninterrupted volcanic tremors of our European world', yet they provide no answer other than compassion and love.

Yet as I consider this, even my appreciation of von Briest's position is brought up short, especially when seen from the perspective of the world after Hitler. I have to wonder whether in a strange way von Briest is not a forerunner of the transformation of the family man Hannah Arendt describes: 'from a responsible member of society, interested in all public affairs, to a "bourgeois" concerned only with his private existence and knowing no civic virtue ...' For it is such a good family man, Arendt argues, who made Nazi mass murders possible by following orders to secure the lives of his wife and children. Seen in this light, the wide field suddenly appears as an evasion of von Briest's own responsibility in his daughter's tragedy since, in the tradition of his class, he married her off to the stodgy and narrow bureaucrat Instetten. And when she rebelled by having a rather desperate affair, Briest refused to question the social system which he himself had affirmed and promoted, and which eventually led to her death. Instead, he hides behind this notion of a wide field.

62

The Partiality of Everything

What times are these ...

In an effort to find my own way through this wide field, treacherous with its hidden mines, I remember lines from one of Bertolt Brecht's poems with the title 'To Those Who Follow in Our Wake':

> *What times are these where*
> *A conversation about trees is almost a crime*
> *Because it includes a silence about so many misdeeds.*

Brecht's theatre on the Schiffbauerdamm was just minutes away from my grandparents' apartment on Luisenstrasse but miles apart from them spiritually. My grandparents did not like Brecht's plays, full of cheating and violent underworld creatures, nor did they sympathise with his radical Marxist politics. I am sure they did not attend the 1928 premiere of *A Three Penny Opera*. Nevertheless, Brecht's poem expresses something that is relevant to my perplexity about Api's life.

A silence that is almost a crime is a chilling spectre that lays its finger on many, if not all, of us and makes innocence impossible. I am reminded again of Martin Luther King's *Letter From Birmingham Jail*, in which he condemned not only the actions of bad people but the silence of the good.

Yet telling Api's story, I did not want to condemn him; I wanted to be one of those who break the silence, sometimes referred to as the Germans' 'second guilt', and recount and account as clearly as I could. I found out that this led to unwelcome discoveries and an uncomfortable questioning of my family history. But it also brought up little kernels of insight from the buried past. For me the balance adds up to an inconvenient past which will always remain fragmentary and to a large extent unrecoverable.

In this way, Api's story not only raises disturbing questions about myself and my family, but it also helps to stitch together some sense of history. 'There exists no position within an epoch from where one can view the history of that epoch,' Goethe once wrote. 'Indeed,' added Ernst von Salomon in his novel *The Questionnaire*, 'there was only a personal position, and only the sum of reports from such positions had to be the material in unlimited amounts for writing history since "truth lies partially in everything".' I might be so bold to add that truth lies in 'the partiality of everything'. In this way my love, my partiality, for my grandfather and the open questions and partial truths become part of a fabric of history.

In the end, when I am left with many explanations but no complete answer, is it too glib and simple-minded to conclude that compassion and love, or call it partiality, should not be selective and cannot be separated from any accounting and recounting of Api's story and of history? If we accept the notion that we are all responsible for the acts of our government, that we are all politically guilty, we need to learn to become more humane toward all around us and learn to forgive others as well as ourselves. This does not release even my post-war generation from being accountable for what was done during the Third Reich and living with that history. But if love and compassion can help us understand, though not excuse, what happened to people like my grandfather, then perhaps they can help us see and accept our common humanity and appreciate how it binds us all together across nationality, race or gender. A belief in, and commitment to, this common humanity might help us to prevent any repetition of the traumas of the twentieth century.

In Api's poems from the post-war years, love and compassion feature prominently. I remember a line from his Christmas poem of 1952 that I had to recite when I was 10. It says that 'Love is man's most beautiful strength'. In view of the crimes of the Nazi regime, and the horrors of two world wars and its millions of dead, the question still remains whether this is wisdom or evasion. Does it show a Panglossian resignation and denial of responsibility or a profound understanding of life through humanity and compassion? I am afraid I still cannot find any solid ground upon which to stand in this 'wide field'.

Source Notes

2 You Made Soap out of my Aunt

'was a prize specimen of German self-contempt' Mann, *Dr. Faustus*, p. 59.
'To do this is to condemn your ancestors!' Ball, p. 63.

3 A Clash of Memories

'Decisions that influence the course of history' Haffner, p. 183.
'by retelling my private, unimportant story' Haffner, p. 182.
'Behind and amid all great events' Stafford, p. xiv.
'The guilt felt about the Holocaust' Grayling, p. 115.
'The descendants of the bombed' Grayling, pp. 1–2.
'the importance of individual historical experience' Anderson, p. 38.
'We will have to repent' King, p. 92.
'We're not responsible for what our ancestors did' Ball, p. 416.

4 Growing Up Prussian

'each one of us has been churned up' Zweig, p. 7.

'media monarch' Clark, p. 589.
'What a man has drawn' Zweig, p. 18.

5 Seven Kilometres of Documents

Statistics in Schmidt, p. 14.
'of thorough knowledge' Schmidt, p. 72.

6 The Shot Heard Around the World

'We saw war as an opportunity' Morton, p. 10.

7 Track 17

'No other nation' Haffner, pp. 52–3.
'The fundamental quality of the disaster' Otto Friedrich, p. 126.

8 Better Times

Statistics of physicians' gross income in 1929, in Kater, p. 260.
'Along the entire Kurfürstendamm' Zweig, p. 359.
'the entire nation' Zweig, p. 360.

9 May Day, May Day, May Day

'turbulent instincts' Domarus (I, 1), p. 192.

'the marriage between' Domarus (I, 1), p. 227.

'no excitement, no hurrahs' Shirer in Noakes (ed.), p. 510.

'You may call me Meier' Read and Fisher, p. 53.

10 Wedding Bells

'Jewish vagabondism' Mosse, p. 72.

'there was a scent of disaster' Read and Fisher, p. 86.

11 Little Noodle

'as completely insane' Osterkamp, p. 369.

'11:27 attack' Kriegstagebuch (III, 1), p. 593.

12 Christmas Trees

'No other Second World War bombing' Middlebrook, p. 306.

'From Alexanderplatz to the Zoo' Benn, p. 353.

'A gargantuan force' Mackinnon, pp. 194–5.

'an overture to the play about hell' Boree, p. 33.

RAF losses, Middlebrook, pp. 306–7.

14 A Death in Prague

'Stalingrad is burned down' Grossmann, p. 125.

16 Russians at the Gates

'Politics!' Bahm, p. 113.

'Berlin itself is no longer a particularly important objective' Bahm, p. 31.

'powerful and full-blooded thrust' Bahm, p. 25.

18 Blocked on All Sides

'The path which we now entered' Schenck, p. 140.

20 Mood Reports

'Berliner! Haltet aus' Beevor, p. 315.

'The bombs have shattered my churches' in Price, title page.

'The situation looks bad' Wette (ed.), p. 259.

'In the center of Berlin that night' Beevor, p. 366.

21 Humans are Fiercer

Losses of Operation Berlin, Le Tissier, p. 225.

'Was she fierce?' Beevor, p. 394.

'The tanks are so covered in flowers' Beevor, p. 395.

'Twenty-three soldiers' Kardoff, p. 217.

22 You Not Lie

'The Führer has died' Kriegstagebuch (IV, 2), p. 1274.

'Every hour that you continue' Rürup, p. 37.

'In this difficult hour' Kriegstagebuch (IV, 2), p. 1282.

23 My Painful Hour

Berlin Mitte alone had 127 million cubic feet of rubble, Bahm, p. 48.

27 The Silence

'I have not found a single German' Stafford, p. 506.

29 Professional Development

'hardly be overrated' Stafford, p. 136.

35 Without the Faintest Guilt

'The Germans have only themselves to blame' Stafford, p. 129.

'Don't get chummy with Jerry' Stafford,
p. 128.
'the main purpose of the ban' Stafford,
p. 130.

36 The Allies are Coming
'a continuation of Nazi-sanctioned'
A. Grossmann, p. 200.

40 We'd be Lucky to get Ike Cleared
'The Americans insisted that
de-Nazification' MacDonogh, p. 243.
'It was only once the properly
completed questionnaire'
MacDonogh, p. 348.
'Americans handled almost 170,000'
MacDonogh, p. 355.
'De-Nazification. Those guys' Kanon,
p. 265.
'as fleeting as the moment' v. Salomon,
p. 52.
'How can I understand the
questionnaire' v. Salomon, p. 8.
'Today we are not only asked' v.
Salomon, p. 225.

45 A Little Closer to Thee
'The Allies were obsessed' MacDonogh,
p. 347.

58 Trying to Understand
'The two are entirely separate' Röpke,
pp. 140–1.
'May the almighty God' Domarus (I, 1),
p. 194.
'were popular in so far as they were
identified' Fritsche, p. 228.
'If there had been barricades' Mosse,
pp. 367–8.
'The government of today's Germany'
Domarus (I, 2), p. 494.
'To make all Germans responsible'
MacDonogh, p. xiii.

59 And Yet ...
'The brutal terms in which all
nationalists regarded' Fritsche, p. 209.
'It is simply not true to say' Neuhaus,
p. 6.
'If Goldhagen is right' Neuhaus, p. 4.
'Our thinking is usually constrained'
Haffner, pp. 102–3.
'they who were the Nazi's first
accomplices' Arendt, p. 126.
'Hitler's threats were so utterly
implausible' Gay, p. 112.
Hostile questions, see Gay, p. 124.
'While all those formidable
transformations' Churchill, *Great
Contemporaries*, p. 228.
'Those who have met Herr Hitler'
Churchill, *Great Contemporaries*,
p. 232.
'One may dislike Hitler's system'
Churchill, *Step by Step*, pp. 143–4.
'Were England to suffer a national
disaster' Churchill in Jaspers, p. 82.
Journalists Adam LeBor and Roger
Boyes, *Seduced by Hitler*, p. 176.
'For the Berliners of those early years'
Friedrich, pp. 391–2.

60 Inner Emigration
'No one who has not lived for years'
Shirer, *Rise and Fall*, p. 247.
'I myself was to experience' Shirer, *Rise
and Fall*, p. 247.
'It was surprising and sometimes
consternating' Shirer, *Rise and Fall*,
p. 247.
'The first norm which Hitler' Jersak in
Echternkamp, p. 337.
'It was totally impossible to form an
opposition' Wolff-Mönckeberg,
p. 136.
'He who wants to talk and judge
Germany' Benn, p. 388.
'Only he who has lived twelve years under
Nazi terror' MacDonogh, p. 348.

'even politically minded people'
Peukert, p. 77.
'we Germans, every German' Jaspers,
p. 65.
'In view of the crimes' Jaspers, p. 56.
'Germany under the Nazi regime was a
penitentiary' Jaspers, p. 73.
'We did not go into the streets' Jaspers,
p. 65.
'Politically everyone acts in the modern
state' Jaspers, p. 56.
'In how far can a human being' Carole
Stern quoted in v. Arnim, p. 229.
'can be determined only by the One'
Arendt, p. 123.
'Where all are guilty' Arendt, p. 126.
'There are many who share
responsibility' Arendt, p. 125.
'For the idea of humanity' Arendt,
p. 131.
'The thesis of the collective guilt of all
Germans' Röpke, p. 221.

'The lack of understanding' Stafford,
p. 506.
'The German masses seem totally
apolitical' MacDonogh, p. 356.
'The horizon has become narrow'
Jaspers, p. 29.
'German victimhood became incorrect'
Anderson, p. 31.
'Unacknowledged suffering' Anderson,
p. 32.
'the importance of individual historical
experience' Anderson, p. 38.

61 A Wide Field
'from a responsible member of society'
Arendt, p. 129.

62 The Partiality of Everything
'There exists no position' v. Salomon,
p. 391.

Acknowlededgments

The archives of Humboldt University in Berlin provided volumes about my grandfather's career and archivist Ilona Kalb even uncovered as yet unregistered materials. Dr Karin Köhler at the Landeskirchliche Archiv in Berlin helped me to trace Pastor Küssner of the Philippus Apostel Church, Dr Mauersberger's archive for Berlin-Mitte gave much information about the district and its history, and Pastor Ingrid Hamel sent me material about the Charite Chapel. Dr med Manfred Stürzbecher provided information on auxiliary military hospitals. I often relied on Dr John M. Lewis for historical and military information. Finally, I want to thank Eric Myers whose comments on an early version of the book helped me to revisualise it.

I have been lucky to have found Isabel Atherton as my agent. She provided insights which led to a major revision and never failed to help with her enthusiasm and efficiency. Sadly, my mother had already passed away when I started but I have absorbed much from her and my stepfather, Dr Hanns Martin Schoenfeld, filled in some gaps. My son, Dr Benedict Robinson, provided related literature and suggested improvements. But the most indefatigable collaborator was my husband Dr Mike Keen. He spent hours over the drafts and helped me to reorganise. Many of the chapter titles are his as well. Most importantly, he supported me with his love and enthusiasm. It truly was a collaboration.

Bibliography

All the books listed here have helped tremendously to flesh out my account. However, I want to single out two of the most inspiring, insightful sources that have guided me through this personal history: Antony Beevor's *The Fall of Berlin 1945*, which combines a broad historical perspective with illuminating insights into everyday life in Berlin at that time, and Ian Kershaw's renowned two-volume history, which paints both a vast and detailed portrait of Hitler and the Third Reich.

Diaries, Interviews, Eyewitness Reports: Berlin 1945

Andreas-Friedrich, Ruth, *Schauplatz Berlin. Tagebuchaufzeichnungen 1945 bis 1948* (Frankfurt am Main: Suhrkamp, 1984).

Anonymous, *A Woman in Berlin. Eight Weeks in the Conquered City. A Diary* (New York: Henry Holt and Co., 2005. First published in 1953).

Benn, Gottfried, *Briefe an F.W. Oelze 1932–1945* (München: Limes, 1977).

Bielenberg, Christabel, *The Past is Myself* (London: Chatto and Wondus, 1968, Penguin 1989 under title *Christabel*).

Boldt, Gerhard, *Hitler. The Last Ten Days* (New York: Coward, McCann and Geoghegan, 1973. First published in German as *Die letzten Tage der Reichskanzlei*, Rowohlt, 1947).

Boveri, Margret, *Tage des Überlebens. Berlin 1945* (München: R. Piper and Co., 1968).

Diem, Liselott, *Fliehen oder bleiben? Dramatisches Kriegsende in Berlin* (Freiburg: Herder, 1982).

Doernberg, Stefan, *Befreiung 1945. Ein Augenzeugenbericht* (Berlin: Verlag Dietz, 1975).

Ebermayer, Erich, *Denn heute gehört uns Deutschland ... Persönliches und politisches Tagebuch* (Hamburg: Paul Zsolnay, 1959).

Findahl, Theo, *Letzter Akt – Berlin 1939–1945* (Hamburg: Hammerich und Lesser, 1946).

Gay, Peter, *My German Question. Growing Up in Nazi Berlin* (Yale University Press, 1998).

Gosztony, Peter (ed.), *Der Kampf um Berlin 1945 in Augenzeugenberichten* (Düsseldorf: Karl Rauch, 1970).

Haffner, Sebastian, *Defying Hitler* (London: Weidenfeld and Nicolson, 2002).

Höcker, Karla, *Die letzten und die ersten Tage. Berliner Aufzeichnungen 1945* (Berlin: Bruno Hessling, 1966).

Hunt, Irmgard, *On Hitler's Mountain. Overcoming the Legacy of a Nazi Childhood* (New York: Harper Perennial, 2006).

Junge, Traudl, *Until the Final Hour. Hitler's Last Secretary* (Ed. Melissa Müller. New York: Arcade Publishing, 2004).

Kardoff, Ursula von, *Diary of a Nightmare. Berlin 1942–1945* (London: Rupert Hart-Davis, 1965. Originally published in German by Biederstein 1962).

Knoke, Heinz, *Die grosse Jagd. Bordbuch eines deutschen Jagdfliegers* (Rinteln: C. Bösendahl, 1952).

Köhler, Jochen, *Klettern in der Grossstadt. Volkstümliche Geschichten vom Überleben in Berlin 1933–1945* (Berlin: Das Arsenal, 1979).

Koller, Karl, *Der letzte Monat. 14. April bis 27. Mai 1945. Tagebuchaufzeichnugen des ehemaligen Chefs des Genralstabs der deutschen Luftwaffe* (München: Bechtle, 1985).

Lange, Horst, *Tagebücher aus dem Zweiten Weltkrieg* (Hans Dieter Schäfer, ed. Mainz: v. Hase & Koehler, 1979).

Mackinnon, Marianne, *The Naked Years. Growing up in Nazi Germany* (London: Chatto and Windus, 1987).

Menzel, Matthias, *Die Stadt ohne Tod. Berliner Tagebuch 1943/45* (Berlin: Carl Habel, 1946).

Schäfer, Hans Dieter, *Berlin im Zweiten Weltkrieg. Der Untergang der Reichshauptstadt in Augenzeugenberichten* (München: Piper, 1985).

Schenck, Ernst-Günther, *Ich sah Berlin sterben. Als Arzt in der Reichskanzlei* (Herford: Nicolaische Verlagsbuchhandlung, 1970).

Studnitz von, Hans-Georg, *While Berlin Burns. The Diary of Hans-Georg von Studnitz 1943–1945* (London: Weidenfeld and Nicolson, 1964. German ed. *Als Berlin brannte*, Stuttgart: W. Kohlhammer, 1963).

Vassiltchikov, Marie, *Berlin Diaries 1940–1945* (New York: Vintage Books, 1985).

Wolff-Mönckeberg, Mathilde, *On the Other Side. To My Children: From Germany 1940–1945* (London: Peter Owen, 1979).

Selected General Bibilography

Anderson, Mark M., 'Crime and Punishment', *The Nation* (17 October 2005), pp. 32–8.

Arendt, Hannah, 'Organized Guilt and Universal Responsibility', *Essays in Understanding 1930–1954* (New York: Schocken Books, 1994), pp. 121–32.

Arnim, Gabriele von, *Das grosse Schweigen. Von der Schwierigkeit, mit dem Schatten der Vergangenheit zu leben* (München: Kindler, 1989).

Ball, Edward, *Slaves in the Family* (New York: Ballantine, 1998).

Beck, Earl R., *Under the Bombs. The German Homefront 1942–1945* (University of Kentucky Press, 1986).

Beevor, Antony, *The Fall of Berlin 1945* (Penguin, 2002).

Bengt von zur Mühlen, *Der Todeskampf der Reichshauptstadt* (Berlin-Kleinmachnow: Chronos, 1994).

Bessel, Richard (ed.), *Life in the Third Reich* (Oxford University Press, 1987).

Boree, Karl Friedrich, *Frühling 1945. Chronik einer Berliner Familie* (Darmstadt: Franz Schneekluth, 1954).

Borkowski, Dieter, *Wer weiss, ob wir uns wiedersehen. Erinnerungen an eine Berliner Jugend* (Frankfurt am Main: S. Fischer, 1980).

Braumüller, Maximilian, *Geschichte des Königin Augusta Garde-Grenadier Regiments Nr. 4* (Berlin: Ernst Siegfried Mittler und Sohn, 1901).

Brunner, Claudia and Uwe von Seltmann, *Schweigen die Täter, reden die Enkel* (Frankfurt/Main: Fischer, 2006).

Burkert, Hans-Norbert, Matussek, Klaus, and Obschernitzki, Doris (eds), *Zerstört Besiegt Befreit. Der Kampf um Berlin bis zur Kapitulation 1945* (Berlin: Stätten der Geschichte Berlins, Band 7, 1985).

Childers, Thomas, *The Nazi Voter. The Social Foundations of Fascism in Germany, 1919–1933* (University of North Carolina Press, 1983).

Churchill, Winston, *Great Contemporaries* (New York: G.P. Putnam's Sons, 1937).

———, *Step by Step 1936–1939* (New York: Putnam's, 1939).

Clark, Christopher, *Iron Kingdom. The Rise and Downfall of Prussia, 1600–1947* (Harvard University Press, 2006).

Diehl, James M., *Paramilitary Politics in Weimar Germany* (Indiana University Press, 1977).

Dinter, Andreas, *Berlin in Trümmern. Ernährungslage und medizinische Versorgung der Bevölkerung Berlins nach dem II. Weltkrieg* (Berlin: Frank Wünsche, 1999).

Döhring, Bruno D., *Mein Lebensweg. Zwischen den Vielen und der Einsamkeit* (Gütersloh: Bertelsmann, 1952).

Domarus, Max (ed.), *Hitler: Reden und Proklamationen 1932–1945* (Würzburg: Schmidt, 1962–63).

313

Echternkamp, Jörg (ed.), *Germany and the Second World War*, Vol. IX/I. *German Wartime Society 1939–1945* (Oxford: Clarendon Press, 2008).

Engelmann, Bernt, *Berlin. Eine Stadt wie keine andere* (München: Bertelsmann, 1986).

Falconer, Jonathan, *The Bomber Command Handbook 1939–1945* (Sutton, 1998).

Friedrich, Jörg, *Der Brand. Deutschland im Bombenkrieg 1940–1945* (München: Propyläen, 2002).

Friedrich, Otto, *Before the Deluge. A Portrait of Berlin in the 1920s* (New York: HarperCollins, 1972).

Fritsche, Peter, *Germans into Nazis* (Harvard University Press, 1998).

Giordano, Ralph, *Die zweite Schuld oder von der Last Deutscher zu sein* (Hamburg: Rasch und Röhring Verlag, 1987).

Goerke, Heinz, *Die Militärärztlichen Bildungsanstalten von ihrer Gründung bis zur Gegenwart* (Zürich: Edition Olms 1986. Reprint of edition Berlin 1895).

Goldhagen, Daniel Jonah, *Hitler's Willing Executioners. Ordinary Germans and the Holocaust* (New York: Vintage Books, 1997).

Grayling, A.C., *Among the Dead Cities* (New York: Walker and Co., 2006).

Grossmann, Atina, 'The Debate Will Not End: The Politics of Abortion in Germany from Weimar to National Socialism and the Postwar Period', in Manfred Berg and Geoffrey Cocks (eds), *Medicine and Modernity: Public Health and Medical Care in 19th and 20th Century Germany* (Cambridge University Press, 1997), pp. 193–212.

Grossmann, Vasily, *A Writer at War. A Soviet Journalist with the Red Army 1941–1945* (New York: Vintage Books, 2005).

Isherwood, Christian, *Mr. Norris Changes Trains* and *Goodbye Berlin*.

Italiaander, Rolf, Bauer, Arnold and Krafft, Herbert (eds), *Berlins Stunde Null* (Düsseldorf: Droste, 1979).

Jameson, Egon, *Berlin so wie es war* (Düsseldorf: Droste, 1969).

Jansen, Christian, Lutz Niethammer and Bernd Weisbrod (eds), *Von der Aufgabe der Freiheit. Politische Verantwortung und bürgerliche Gesellschaft im 19. und 20. Jahrhundert* (Berlin: Akademie, 1995).

Japsers, Karl, *Die Schuldfrage* (Heidelberg: Lambert Schneider, 1946).

Kannapin, Norbert, *Die deutsche Feldpostübersicht 1939–1945* (3 vols) (Osnabrück, Biblio, 1980–82).

Kanon, Joseph, *The Good German* (New York: Henry Holt, 2001).

Kater, Michael H., *Doctors Under Hitler* (The University of North Carolina Press, 1989).

———, *The Nazi Party. A Social Profile of Members and Leaders 1919–1945* (Harvard University Press, 1983).

Kershaw, Ian, *Hitler 1889–1936: Hubris* (New York: W.W. Norton, 1999); and *1936–45: Nemesis* (New York: W.W. Norton, 2000).

Bibliography

Kettenacker, Lothar (ed.), *Ein Volk von Opfern?* (Berlin: Rowohlt, 2003).

King, Martin Luther Jr, *I Have a Dream. Writings and Speeches that Changed the World* (HarperSanFrancisco, 1992).

Kiaulehn, Walther, *Berlin. Schicksal einer Weltstadt* (München: Biederstein, 1958).

Kraatz, Helmut, *Zwischen Klinik und Hörsaal* (Berlin: Verlag der Nation, 1977).

Kronika, Jacob, *Der Untergang Berlins*. (Flensburg: Christian Wolf, 1946).

LeBor, Adam and Roger Boyes, *Seduced by Hitler* (Naperville, IL: Sourcebooks, Inc., 2001).

Le Tissier, Tony, *The Battle of Berlin 1945* (New York: St Martin's Press, 1988).

MacDonogh, Giles, *After the Reich. From the Fall of Vienna to the Berlin Airlift* (London: John Murray, 2007).

Madison, James H., *What We've Learned about World War II* (Indiana University Institute for Advanced Study, 2006).

Mann, Heinrich, *Der Untertan* (Berlin: Claasen, 1958).

Mann, Thomas, *Dr. Faustus* (Berlin: Suhrkamp, 1947).

Middlebrook, Martin, *The Berlin Raids. RAF Bomber Command Winter 1943–44* (London: Viking, 1988).

Morton, Frederic, *Thunder at Twilight. Vienna 1913/1914* (Cambridge, MA: Da Capo Press, 2001).

Mosse, George L., *Nazi Culture. Intellectual, Cultural and Social Life in the Third Reich* (New York: Grosset and Dunlap, 1966).

Nelson, Walter Henry, *The Berliners. Their Saga and their City* (New York: David McKay Company, 1969).

Neuhaus, Richard John, 'Daniel Goldhagen's Holocaust', in *First Things* (65, Aug–Sept 1996).

Noakes, Jeremy (ed.), *Nazism 1919–1945* (Vol. 4), *The German Home Front in World War II, A Documentary Reader* (University of Exeter Press, 1998).

Osterkamp, Theo, *Durch Höhen und Tiefen jagt ein Herz* (Heidelberg: Kurt Vowinckel, 1952).

Pehle, Walter H. (ed.), *Der historische Ort des Nationalsozialismus* (Frankfurt/Main: Fischer, 1990).

Pehle, Walter H. and Wolfgang Benz (eds), *Encyclopedia of German Resistance to the Nazi Movement* (New York: Continuum, 1997).

Pem, *Heimweh nach dem Kurfürstendamm*.

Plievier, Theodor, *Berlin* (München: Kurt Desch, 1954).

Peukert, Detlev J.K., *Inside Nazi Germany. Conformity, Opposition, and Racism in Everyday Life* (Yale University Press, 1987. Original German edition 1982).

Price, Alfred, *Blitz on Britain. The Bomber Attacks on the United Kingdom 1939–1945* (London: Ian Halland, 1977).

Read, Anthony and Fisher, David, *The Fall of Berlin* (New York: W.W. Norton, 1993).

Rein, Heinz, *Finale Berlin* (Berlin: JHW Dietz Nachf., no date).

Richie, Alexandra, *Faust's Metropolis. A History of Berlin* (New York: Carroll and Graf, 1998).

Röpke, Wilhelm, *The Solution of the German Problem* (New York: G.P. Putnam's Sons, 1946).

Rürup, Reinhard (ed.), *Berlin 1945. Eine Dokumentation* (Berlin: Verlag Willmuth Arenhövel, 2nd improved ed., 1995).

Ryan, Cornelius, *The Last Battle* (London: Collins, 1966).

Salomon, Ernst von, *Der Fragebogen* (Hamburg: Rowohlt, 1951).

Schmidt, Hermann, *Die Kaiser Wilhelm Akademie für das militärärztliche Bildungswesen von 1895 bis 1910* (Zürich: Edition Olms, 1995, reprint of 1910).

Schoeps, Julius. H., Ein *Volk von Mördern?* (Hamburg: Hoffmann und Campe, 1996).

Schramm, Percy Ernst, *Kriegstagebuch des Oberkommandos der Wehrmacht*, Vols 1–4 (Frankfurt/Main: Bernard und Graefe Verlag für Wehrwesen, 1961–65).

Schultz-Naumann, Joachim, *The Last Thirty Days, the War Diary of the German Armed Forces High Command from April to May 1945* (Lanham, Maryland: Madison Books, 1991).

Sebald, W.G., *On the Natural History of Destruction* (New York: Random House, 2003).

Senfft, Alexandra, *Schweigen tut weh. Eine deutsche Familiengeschichte* (Berlin: Ullstein, 2008).

Serge, Victor, *Unforgiving Years*. Translated by Richard Greeman (New York: New York Review Books, 2008).

Shirer, William L., *The Rise and Fall of the Third Reich* (New York: Simon and Schuster, 1960).

———, *End of a Berlin Diary* (New York: Alfred A. Knopf, 1947).

Sichrovsky, Peter, *Schuldig Geboren. Kinder aus Nazifamilien* (Kiepenheuer und Witsch, 1987).

Singer, Peter, *Pushing Time Away* (New York: Ecco, 2004).

Slowe, Peter and Woods, Richard, *Battlefield Berlin. Siege, Surrender and Occupation, 1945* (London: Robert Hale, 1988).

Stafford, David, *Endgame, 1945. The Missing Final Chapter of World War II* (New York: Little Brown and Co., 2007).

Steinhoff, Johannes, Pechel, Peter, and Showalter, Dennis (eds), *Deutsche im Zweiten Weltkrieg. Zeitzeugen sprechen* (München: Schneekluth, 1989).

Studier, Manfred, *Der* Corpsstudent *als Idealbild der Wilhelminischen Ära. Untersuchungen zum Zeitgeist 1888–1914* (PhD Dissertation, Friedrich Alexander

University, Erlangen, 1965).

Surminski, Arno, *Vaterland ohne Väter* (Berlin: Ullstein, 2004).

Trampe, Gustav (ed.), *Die Stunde Null. Erinnerungen an Kriegsende und Neuanfang* (Stuttgart: Deutsche Verlags-Anstalt, 1995).

Trevor-Roper, H.R., *The Last Days of Hitler* (New York: Macmillan, 1947).

Werner, Bruno E., *Die Zwanziger Jahre* (München: F. Bruckmann, 1962).

Wette, Wolfram, Bremer, Ricarda, and Vogel, Detlef (eds), *Das letzte halbe Jahr. Stimmungsberichte der Wehrmachtpropaganda 1944/45* (Essen: Klartext, 2001).

Williamson, Murray, *Strategy for Defeat. The Luftwaffe 1933–1945* (Maxwell Air Force Base, Alabama: Air University Press, 1983).

Wippermann, Wolfgang, *Wessen Schuld? Vom Historikerstreit zur Goldhagen-Kontroverse* (Berlin: Elefanten Press, 1997).

Zweig, Stefan, *Die Welt von Gestern. Erinnerungen eines Europäers* (Berlin: S. Fischer, 1982).

Index